Healing Power of Breathing

TARIT KUMAR PAL

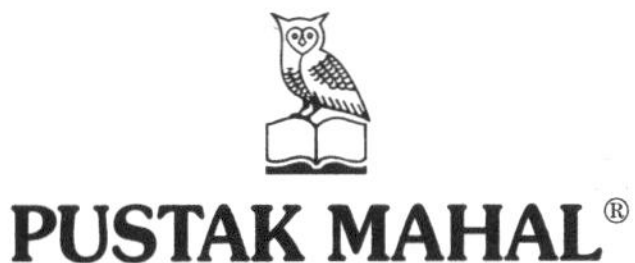

PUSTAK MAHAL®

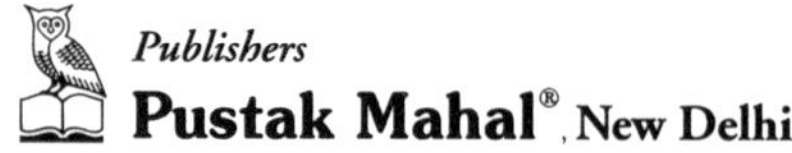

Administrative office and sale centre

J-3/16, Daryaganj, New Delhi-110002
☎ 23276539, 23272783, 23272784 • *Fax:* 011-23260518
E-mail: info@pustakmahal.com • *Website:* www.pustakmahal.com

Branches

Bengaluru: ☎ 080-22234025 • *Telefax:* 080-22240209
E-mail: pustakmahalblr@gmail.com
Mumbai: ☎ 022-22010941, 022-22053387
E-mail: rapidex@bom5.vsnl.net.in
Patna: ☎ 0612-3294193 • *Telefax:* 0612-2302719
E-mail: rapidexptn@rediffmail.com

ISBN 978-81-223-1561-5

Edition: 2015

*Printed at : **Radha Offset, Delhi***

'Healing Power of breathing' is dedicated to my Gurudev late Shri Subhash Chakraborty, my father late Shri Hemendra Nath Pal, my mother late Shrimati Sujala Pal and my friend late Sri Ram Chakraborty.

Acknowledgement

I am deeply indebted to my wife Srimati Urmimala Pal for not only patiently tolerating but also encouraging me during the entire period of my compilation of the book. My grandson Sriman Prodyot Khandai as usual was the positive push behind my efforts all the time. I express my sincere thanks to the silent background support of my daughter Dr. Tanusree Khandai and son-in-law Dr. Nishikkanta Khandai. They updated my knowledge on computer applications from time to time which helped me immensely in my compilation work. I also express my gratitude to the publisher for the cover design of the book.

Supporting sketches (figures) are all collected from free circulation of leaflets during my Gurudev's discussions in our Arrah Village ashram at Durgapur, free available images in internet and some medical books and journals. Though I am grateful to all the sources, I am unable to express my gratitude to any specific person/persons.

Lastly I shall fail in my duty if I do not express my gratitude to my brother-in- law Dr. Shubhomoy Dutta Choudhury and Kriyaban (Kriya Yoga) colleagues late Sri Ram Chakraborty, Sri Asit Bhattacharjee, Sri Tapan Kumar Gupta and Sri Bidyut Ghosh with whom I had discussions on various subjects that feature in the book.

Prologue

On 8th April 2004, me and my wife visited Late Sri Sri Subhash Chakraborty in his residence at Durgapur along with our family friend late Sri Ram Chakraborty and his wife. While we spent around two hours with him, he mostly did the bulk of the talking. He talked on various aspects mostly surrounding human breath. That day I was moved by the depth of his spontaneous talk. While I could feel and understand part of his deliberations, rest of his conveyed messages which apparently appeared to be exciting but beyond my understanding, I carried them in my memory. I could absorb those messages with the blessings of my Gurudev in later years. The gist of the messages that he conveyed that day was, "Breath is your most valuable asset. It is not simply an act of air intake and carbon dioxide elimination only. In fact, breathing is the way of life. If you make proper use of the breath, you can exercise control in your life. It is through the merging of sattvik way of life and proper application of specific breathing practices that you can know your true self". He eventually became my Gurudev. I took diksha from him and became his disciple in the same month.

When my first book on motivation - 'Wake up and make it happen' was published in 2010, my Gurudev went through it and gave me lot of suggestions and advised me to continue writing books on the awareness of various aspects of life for the easy understanding and benefit of the common people, especially the younger generations. Before my second book on motivation 'Power of thoughts' came out in prints in 2013, Gurudev had left us for heavenly abode. Immediately, I decided to compile a write up on the awareness of the different facets of 'breathing'. This is how "Healing power of breathing" took its shape in the form of a book. The book written in three parts concentrates on

1. awareness of human breathing,
2. awareness of prana and how it relates to human breathing.
3. awareness of breathing and prana in spiritual journey.

Though certain common breathing practices are discussed here and there in the book, it is suggested to the prospective readers that all 'specific breathing practices' referred be learned and practiced under the guidance of a teacher with proven credentials.

The first part of the book titled 'HUMAN BREATH' deals with the awareness of basic components of breathing, the respiratory tracts, the mechanism of oxygen absorption, carbon dioxide elimination, various parameters of breathing, the breathing potential, different types of breathing and their effects on human life, influence of breathing on human emotions, importance of postures in different types of breathing practices etc.

The second part titled 'BREATH & PRANA' deals with the awareness of prana and how breath relates to prana. Prana, the vital energy is drawn into the human body through breathing. Although closely related to the air a person breathes in, prana is more subtle than air or oxygen. It is via nadis and chakras that the prana flows in the pranic body. Breath distributes prana as vayus to different parts of the subtle pranic body. Nadis and chakras are the subtle passage ways and distribution junctions of the prana vayus. When the flow of prana vayus through the nadis and chakras are uniform, a person enjoys a good heath, both physically as well as mentally. By adapting specific breathing practices, uniformity of flow of prana vayus through nadis and chakras can be ensured.

The third part of the book titled 'BREATH, PRANA & SPIRITUALITY' deals with the awareness of how breathing spreads prana in the body and leads a person towards journey in the spiritual path. For a person's spiritual journey to commence, it is mandatory that the nadis (carriers of prana) get purified i.e. freed from any blockages, the chakras get activated and the kundalini shakti, the dormant energy gets awakened. All these can be achieved by adapting specific breathing practices in identified asanas along with chanting of guru mantras. When sattvik way of life merges with specific breathing practices to purify, activate and awaken the nadis, chakras and the kundalini shakti respectively, a person heads towards spiritual consciousness.

INDEX

PART ONE: HUMAN BREATH

PART TWO: BREATH & PRANA

PART ONE

HUMAN BREATH

Breathing is a natural phenomenon; nobody can live without it. After birth, human life starts on earth with the first breath a person takes and ends with his last breath before death. In between, there is no stopping. Since irrespective of circumstances and state of being, a person breathes all the time, there is a general tendency for him to take this phenomenon for granted till he experiences breathlessness, reduced vitality, immunity to diseases and emotional instability. When this happens, the person is made aware of the importance of learning about

1. the breathing phenomenon,
2. the detailed respiratory tract,
3. the act of breathing,
4. the mechanism of oxygen absorption in the body,
5. different types of breathing,
6. importance of deep breathing
7. the breath and its influences on emotion.

There is a strong linkage between breath and emotion which generally goes unnoticed to a person even though he himself experiences and sees others experiencing the same every day. Though breathing is a unique involuntary bodily function, it can be made to function voluntarily when a person consciously decides to do so. When the breathing is brought under a person's direct control, he can use it as a tool to influence the mind under different circumstances and bring about over all improvements in the quality of his life.

01. NORMAL BREATHING

After birth, human life starts on earth, with the first breath a person takes and ends with his last breath before death; in between, there is no stopping. Irrespective of circumstances and state of being, a person breathes all the time, there is a general tendency for him to accept it as an involuntary function and take this phenomenon for granted till he experiences-

1. shortness of breath,
2. tightness of chest with feelings of suffocation,
3. jerky breathing often causing sobbing or sighing,
4. quick and rapid breathing,
5. uneven breathing like rapid breathing alternating with long or jerky pause,
6. breathing through mouth even when the nostrils are open,
7. long pause between two breaths signaling as if he is not interested for his next breath,
8. unusual noises while breathing.

When this happens, a person is made aware of the breathing phenomenon, the components of breathing, the respiratory tract, the act and the maximum potential of his breathing. The person is further made aware that even though breathing apparently is an involuntary function, if he desires, he can consciously make voluntary changes in his breathing rhythm for his own physical and mental well being.

02. CYCLE OF A BREATH

The breathing phenomenon has two components - inhalation and exhalation. Drawing of air inside the body from atmosphere is called inhalation or inspiration and discharging of the carbon dioxide rich air from the body back to the atmosphere is called exhalation or expiration.

Inhalation followed by exhalation completes a cycle of normal breath. The duration of each such cycle of breath varies from person to person depending on the type of breathing practice he adapts – slow, medium or fast.

During inhalation, air enters the body through nasal/oral cavity, moves through the back of the mouth above the throat and then through it into the lungs passing on the way number of passageways like trachea, bronchi, bronchioles and finally end up in microscopic air sacs called alveoli. At alveoli which share common walls with the surrounding deoxygenated blood capillaries, the blood capillaries pick up oxygen from the air inhaled. The oxygenated blood is then circulated back to the heart. From the deoxygenated blood capillaries, alveoli pick up carbon dioxide and discharge it to the atmosphere during exhalation. The incoming atmospheric air and the outgoing carbon dioxide rich air flow through the same track but move in reverse directions. The details of this track of reference is discussed in sections 06, 07, 08 and 09 of part one.

The expansion and relaxation of the lungs, expansion and relaxation of the rib cage area and upward and downward movement of the abdomen can be felt by a person during inhalation and exhalation respectively. During inhalation, the air fills the chest cavity. The chest cavity gets emptied out during exhalation. The extent to which the chest cavity is filled during inhalation and subsequently evacuated during exhalation determines the quality of a person's breath. If the breath fills only the top layer of the chest, then the breath is shallow. When the lower chest expands, it signals the filling of the whole chest cavity – an ideal breathing practice that signals maximum intake of air. The lungs capacity are utilized most during belly breathing (discussed in section 16 of part one).

People generally breathe shallow in situations like

1. when they get involved in an argument,
2. when they have too much of work to do,
3. when they are upset over something, and so forth.

There however are many people who regularly breathe shallow because of their life styles. They breathe shallow mainly because of the increasing stress of their modern day living. They are in hurry most of the time; their movements and breathing also follow the same pattern. They get emotional too easily and often suffer from worries and anxieties.

When shallow breathing becomes the way of life and is continued for a long stretch of time, it gets associated with release of host of chemicals and starvation of tissues (due to lower intake of oxygen). These often result in chronic health problems. The good news however is, a person can switch from chest breathing to belly breathing with associated benefits (discussed in section 16 of part one) and adapt different breathing practices to bring the disturbed mind under control in different circumstances (discussed in section 51 of part three).

03. MAJOR ACTIVITIES DURING A BREATH

Two major activities that take place in the body during a cycle of breath are oxygen absorption and carbon dioxide elimination. During inhalation, the air that enters the human body has around 20.95 % oxygen, .038 % carbon dioxide and balance nitrogen. The exhaled air has 5 % carbon dioxide and the rest is nitrogen.

It transpires from above that during every cycle of breathing, the human body absorbs oxygen from the inhaled air, and releases carbon dioxide which is many fold higher than the amount of the carbon dioxide of the inhaled air. The following accounts for the additional carbon dioxide involved during exhalation.

Human heart pumps blood and circulates it to different parts of the body through arteries, arterioles and capillaries. As the blood moves through the body and reaches the capillaries, the surrounding tissues consume oxygen from the blood stream through the process of metabolism and release carbon dioxide into it as a byproduct. This additional carbon dioxide is transferred from the capillaries to the alveoli through the process of gas exchange (explained in section 10 & section11 of part one). From the alveoli, the carbon dioxide rich air is then driven out to the atmosphere during exhalation.

Oxygen is the most critical and vital element for human survival. A person can survive for weeks without food, for days without water but he cannot survive without oxygen even for a few minutes. The chemical basis of energy production in human body is a chemical known as Adenosine Triphosphate (ATP). It has been scientifically established that oxygen is a contributory element towards the production of ATP; in fact, it is the most vital input for production of ATP. When its production goes down, it causes lowered vitality, disease and premature ageing. Some of the major roles played by oxygen in the human body are summarized underneath.

04. ROLE OF OXYGEN IN HUMAN BODY

Intake of oxygen causes purification of the blood stream through the process of gas exchange as explained in section 10 of part one. Oxygen makes the blood cells healthier,

Oxygen activates the entire nervous system. This in turn improves the health of the whole body since the nervous system is connected to every part of the human body.

Oxygen helps the digestive organs to operate more efficiently and also improves the digestion process.

Oxygen is responsible for better integrity in the maintenance of the brain, nerves, glands and other organs of human body. Brain cells in particular are very sensitive to oxygen flow. Occlusion of blood vessels supplying oxygenated blood to the brain cells results in instant death of the brain cells. Cells in the specific areas of the brain are responsible for the movement and functioning of identified parts in the human body. If any specific area of the brain is deprived of oxygen supply due to occlusion of cerebral blood vessels, a person suffers paralysis of the relevant part of the body. This phenomenon is called brain stroke. With ageing, blood vessels get progressively narrowed down because of deposition of various metabolic wastes and loss of elasticity of blood vessel walls etc. This increases the possibility of brain strokes. The above explains why brain strokes are observed more in elderly people.

In the same manner as explained above, if a person's heart muscle is deprived of oxygen because of sudden blockage of coronary vessels supplying oxygenated blood to heart muscles, it results in heart attack.

Oxygen has direct impact on weight control. For those who are overweight, available oxygen helps in burning excess fat. For those who are underweight, available oxygen feeds the starving tissues and glands and brings about improvements.

The benefit of oxygen can be reaped most through intake of maximum oxygen during slow and deep breathing.

05. BENEFITS OF DEEP BREATHING

With conscious deep breathing, the cycle time of a breath is increased. This not only ensures more air (oxygen) to be drawn into the body, it also increases the contact time between the air in the alveoli and blood in the capillaries leading to higher gas exchange in the lungs along with other associated benefits as mentioned below. Some of the benefits associated with deep breathing are listed below.

Deep breathing is the most effective way of toxins removal from the human body. With deep exhalation, one can release up to 70% of the toxins generated in the human body through metabolism. With shallow breathing, other detoxification systems like urination, sweating, feces etc. in the body has to take over charge and work harder to expel waste toxins. This overloads the specific systems of reference and often makes body weaker.

Deep breathing not only increases the amount of oxygen the skin gets, but also increases the flow rate of blood to different parts of the body and thereby slows down the process of ageing. This makes a person look healthier with visible improved skin and reduction in facial wrinkles.

Shallow breathing causes tightening of muscles with associated development of internal stress and anxiety which in turn triggers sympathetic nervous system. Deep breathing is the fastest way to stimulate the parasympathetic nervous system which counters the action of the sympathetic nervous system; it normalizes the brain functions with improved relaxation of mind and reduction in anxiety levels. Function of sympathetic and parasympathetic nervous systems have been discussed in details in section 47.

Deep breathing enhances the elasticity of lungs and rib cage and there by improves breathing capacity.

During deep breathing, the movement of the diaphragm massages the stomach, small intestine, liver and pancreas. Blood circulations in all these organs get stimulated. This improves the health of abdominal and other organs.

With deep breathing, the lungs provide blood with more oxygen; this reduces the amount of work to be done by heart in order to supply oxygenated blood to rest of the body. It also causes a greater pressure differential in the lungs and helps in better circulation of blood. The heart therefore gets little rest and becomes stronger.

In view of the reasons mentioned above, there is no reason why one should not harvest the benefit of deep breathing. Air (oxygen) is a freely available commodity anywhere in the world. No country imposes any tax on its consumption. There however is a limitation to the maximum amount of air that a person can draw in during inhalation; this has been discussed in subsequent sections.

The passageway through which the fresh air moves during inhalation and the carbon dioxide rich air exits during exhalation is known as respiratory tract.

06. RESPIRATORY TRACT

Respiration is derived from the word 'respire' which refers to breathing. When a person respires, he takes in oxygen along with each inhalation and releases carbon dioxide with each exhalation. In terms of biology, respiration is a process in which the cells of an organism obtain energy by combining oxygen and glucose that result in the release of carbon dioxide, water and ATP, the currency of life. The energy freed in the process is used to power the organism's movements and physiological functions.

When a breath is taken, air flows in through the nostrils/mouth. From there through passageways the air passes through the pharynx then through the larynx, down to the trachea. The trachea branches off into two separate streams called bronchi (hollow passageway). Through the primary bronchi the air then passes to the secondary bronchi. From the secondary bronchi air then passes to tertiary bronchi which then passes into the bronchiole. Through the bronchiole the air then moves to terminal bronchiole, then to respiratory bronchiole and finally end up in collections of tiny air sacs individually called an alveolus and collectively known as alveoli. The gas exchange takes place at alveoli. Here the oxygen moves from alveoli to blood capillaries and carbon dioxide moves from blood capillaries to alveoli. Starting from the nasal/oral opening up to the alveoli in the lungs, the entire stretch is known as **respiratory tract**. The carbon dioxide released from alveoli flows through the same tract but moves in opposite direction from the alveoli to the atmosphere via the nose/oral cavity during exhalation.

Respiratory tract is divided into two parts – upper respiratory tract and lower respiratory tract. The lower respiratory tract again is divided into two parts - lower respiratory part 1 and lower respiratory part 2.

07. UPPER RESPIRATORY TRACT

The upper respiratory tract embraces the nasal cavity, oral cavity, pharynx, larynx and the beginning of trachea as shown in figure no. 1.

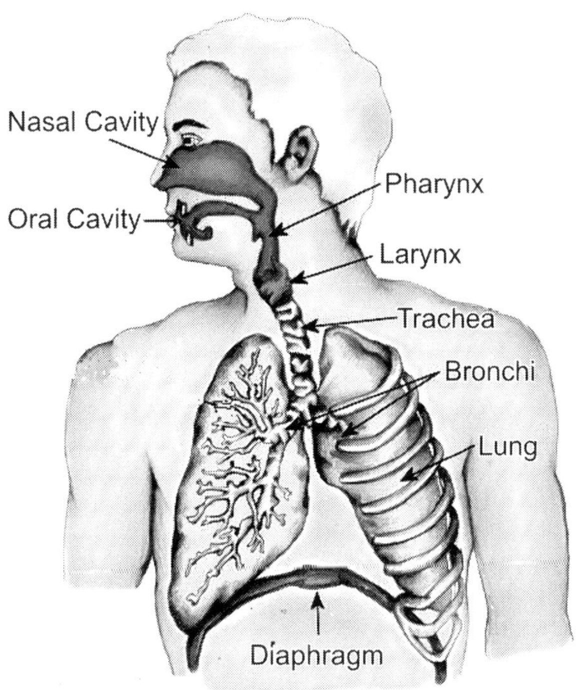

Figure no.1

Nasal and Oral Cavity: They are the openings through which air enters the human body from atmosphere during inhalation and carbon dioxide find exit through exhalation. Inhalation of air through nasal cavity is always advocated as it provides lots of safety mechanisms to the human body and ensures that only fresh air gets entry to the lungs. Some of the striking advantages of breathing through nasal cavity are listed underneath.

1. At the entrance of the nose, there is a screen of hair. It has the capacity to filter and trap dusts, tiny insects and other particles which might be carried in with inhaled air. Entry of air through nose therefore provides a protection to the lungs from injury.
2. Once through the nasal cavity, the air passes along a long passage lined with mucous membranes. Here, if the air is cold, it gets warmed up. If by chance any thin and fine dust particles escape the filter screen of hair mentioned above, it gets arrested here.

3. There are glands in inner nose which can fight with bacilli (microscopic organisms which can cause disease) in case they slip up to this stage.
4. The inner nose contains the olfactory organ through which people sense smell. As per the yogic philosophy, the olfactory organ is believed to be the main absorption point of prana (discussed in part two) in the human body.

The oral cavity is bereft of the above safety mechanisms. Pathogens (micro organism that can cause disease) finding entry into the lungs through mouth breathing can cause serious health problems.

It is not at all difficult to break away from the habit of breathing through the mouth. A person just has to consciously keep his mouth closed and practice breathing through nose; within no time he will automatically develop the habit of breathing through his nose.

Both the above openings join with the pharynx, a hollow passageway.

Pharynx is a hollow and cone shaped passageway connecting the oral and nasal cavities and the larynx. It is commonly known as throat.

Larynx holds the vocal cord. Apart from producing voice, it actively takes part in the process of swallowing and breathing by providing a hollow passageway from the bottom of the pharynx to the top of the trachea. Food and liquids are blocked from entering the opening of the larynx by epiglottis, a flexible flap which acts as a switch between the larynx and the esophagus. Epiglottis permits air to enter the airway to the lungs and food to pass into the gastrointestinal tract. It protects the body from choking on food that would normally obstruct the airway.

Trachea is like a hollow tube. It starts from the larynx and bifurcates into two primary bronchi i.e. smaller hollow tubes.

The bronchi enter the two lungs separately. While one enters the left lung, the other enters the right lung through separate but identical passageways. The trachea connects the upper respiratory tract with the lower respiratory tract part 1 which again is connected to the lower respiratory tract part 2.

08. LOWER RESPIRATORY TRACT PART 1

The **lower respiratory tract part 1** starts from the entry of the primary bronchi to the lungs (left lung and right lung) and runs successively through two separate but identified passageways, joins with **lower respiratory tract 2** and end up in the alveoli in respective lungs.

The **lungs** are a pair of spongy organs where optimum gas exchange between blood and air takes place. Lungs play important role in absorption of oxygen in the human body and elimination of carbon dioxide from the body before it reaches hazardous level.

As the **primary bronchi** starts getting closer to the lung tissues, they progressively branch off to numbers of smaller bronchi which provide passage ways to the inhaled air.

The primary bronchi branch off to numbers of **secondary bronchi**. Each secondary bronchus (singular of bronchi) gives rise to numbers of **tertiary bronchi**. Each tertiary bronchus again branches off into **bronchioles** as shown in figure no. 2.

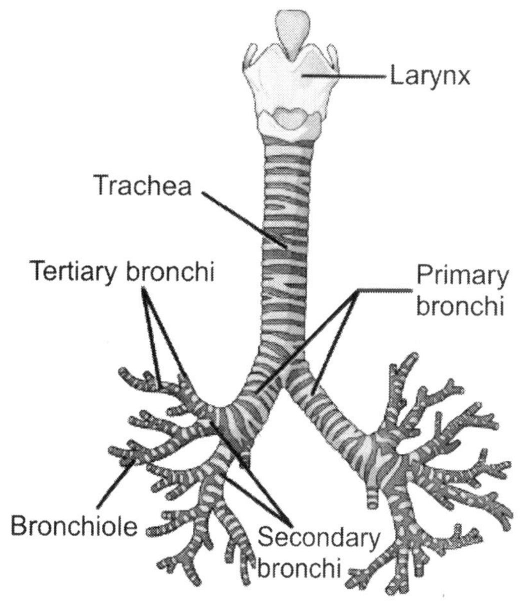

Figure no.2

The bronchioles subsequently get smaller and gets divided into numbers of **terminal bronchioles**.

09. LOWER RESPIRATORY TRACT PART 2

Each terminal bronchiole eventually branches off to form numbers of **respiratory bronchioles**. Respiratory bronchioles are the smallest passageways of the inhaled air to the lungs.

Each respiratory bronchiole finally morph into small collections of air sacs. These air sacs inflate during inhalation of air and deflate during exhalation of carbon dioxide rich air. Individually these air sacs are called **alveolus** and collectively they are known as **alveoli**.

Figure no. 3 illustrates formation of alveolous and alveoli from the respiratory bronchiole. Alveoli resembles bunch of grapes in look.

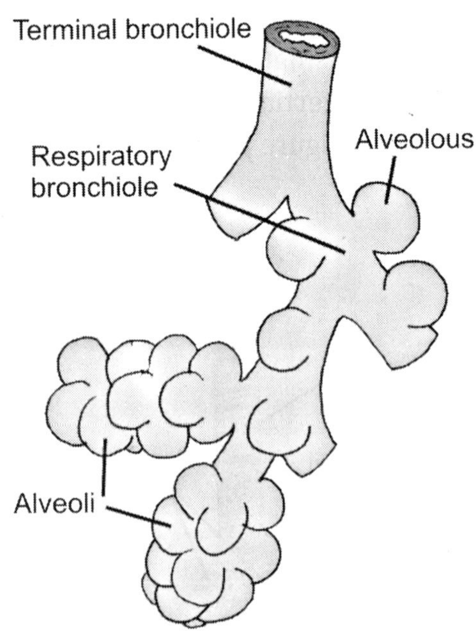

Figure no. 3

Alveoli are very tiny in size but have a very large surface area. It is estimated that lungs contain about 300 million alveoli and their total surface area would be about 70 square meters (which is about

40 times the surface area of the skin). The atmosphere in the alveoli is moist, and the alveoli are surrounded by several number of blood capillaries. The blood capillaries and the alveoli have common walls (commonly known as membranes). The exchange of oxygen and carbon dioxide between the blood capillaries and air in the alveoli occur across these membranes.

10. ATMOSPHERE IN ALVEOLI

It is mentioned above that the atmosphere in the alveoli is moist, and the alveoli are surrounded by several numbers of blood capillaries. It has further been mentioned that the blood capillaries and the alveoli have common walls called membranes and the exchange of oxygen and carbon dioxide between the blood capillaries and air in the alveoli occur across these membranes.

Gas exchange basically is a process where two gases across a membrane move in opposite directions from the area of high concentration to the area of low concentration. This process is also known as a process of diffusion. The process is encouraged most when the participating gases spread over large surface areas in a moist atmosphere.

Both oxygen and carbon dioxide (a by product of body's metabolism) dissolve in blood and are transported around the human body through blood vessels. Heart pumps and supplies oxygenated blood through **arteries** to different parts of the body. Each artery branches off to number of **arterioles** and arteriole again branches off to numbers of capillaries. **Capillaries** are the smallest blood carrying vessels in the body. Blood coming out of the heart while flowing through different parts of the body get progressively deoxygenated as the surrounding cells and tissues consume oxygen. As the cells use the oxygen, carbon dioxide produced due to body's metabolism gets absorbed into the blood stream. That is why the bloods in the capillaries which reach alveoli have lower concentration of oxygen with higher concentration of carbon dioxide. The alveoli on the other hand always have continuous supply of oxygen because of intake of fresh air with every inhalation.

The atmosphere prevailing in alveoli as mentioned above satisfies all the conditions for gas exchange to take place.

11. OXYGEN & CARBON DIOXIDE EXCHANGE

In the most conducive atmosphere for diffusion, gas exchange takes place between the oxygen of alveoli and carbon dioxide of the blood capillaries in the following manner.

1. Oxygen from the alveoli moves across the membranes (walls between the alveoli and the surrounding blood capillaries) to the blood capillaries,
2. carbon dioxide moves across the membranes in opposite directions (from the blood capillaries to alveoli in the lungs).

Due to the above gas exchange mechanism, the deoxygenated capillary blood again gets oxygenated. It then flows through venules and subsequently through veins and goes back to heart for recirculation. Venule and vein are blood carriers. The carbon dioxide which gets transferred to the alveoli in the respiratory tract, subsequently finds exit to the atmosphere during exhalation.

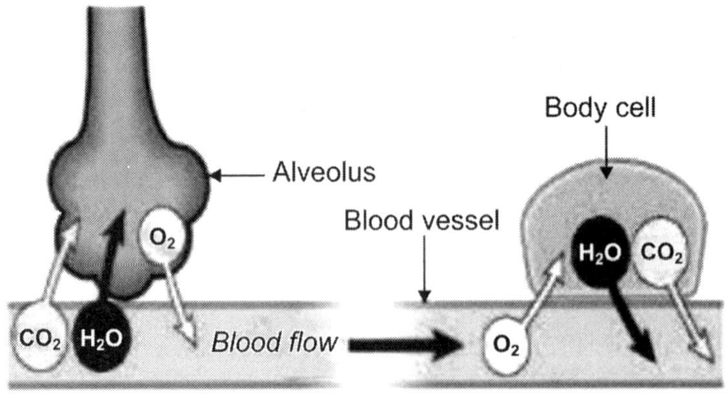

Figure no. 4.

Figure no. 4 illustrates the process of

1. gas exchange that takes place across the membranes which separates the flow of blood and air in the capillary and alveoli respectively,

2. deoxygenetion of blood vessels with absorption of carbon dioxide.

The summary of the events of respiration is shown in table no. 1.

SUMMARY OF THE EVENTS OF RESPIRATION
1. Breathing: Breathing air into & out of the lungs.
2. External respiration: Exchange of gases between the air in the alveoli in the lungs & blood in the capillaries.
3. Gas transport by blood: Transport of oxygen to the body cells & the return of carbon dioxide back to the blood vessel.
4. Internal respiration: Exchange of gases between the blood & the body cells.
5. Cellular respiration: Oxygen in the body cell is used to convert nutrients into adenosine phosphate with carbon dioxide and water. Energy released in the process is utilized in the functioning of different human organs.

Table no. 1

12. ACT OF BREATHING

It has been shown in figure no. 1, that below the lungs there is a dome shaped structure of muscles and fibrous tissues known as **diaphragm**. Though not a part of the respiratory tract, diaphragm plays an active role in the act of breathing. The diaphragm separates the thoracic (chest) and abdominal cavities.

During inhalation, when the diaphragm contracts the dome flattens and moves downward into the abdominal cavity. This movement increases the thoracic cavity; the increase being directly proportional to the extent of the 'movement' of reference. The diaphragm contraction also induces the lower ribs to move upward and forward, which further increases the thoracic volume. This increase of volume lowers the air pressure in the alveoli to below atmospheric pressure. Because air always flows from a region of high pressure to a region of lower pressure, atmospheric air rushes in through the respiratory tract and into the alveoli.

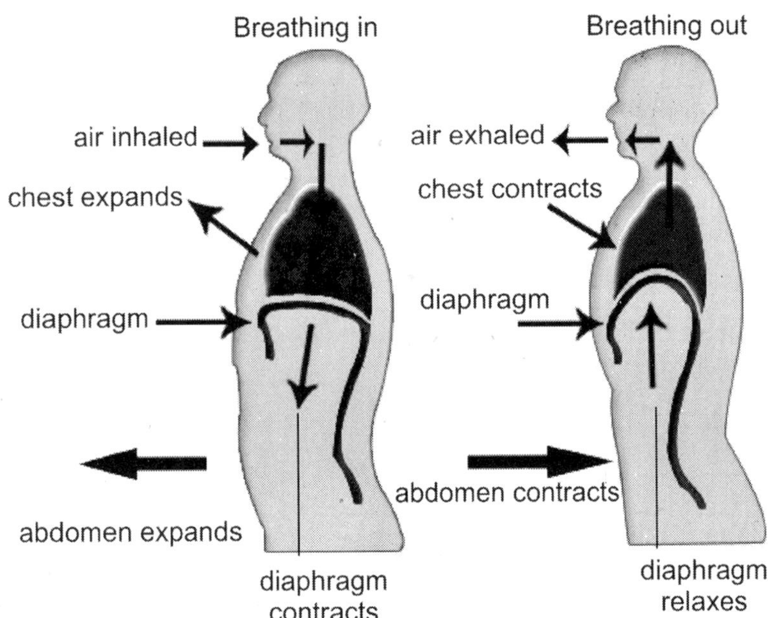

Figure no. 5

During exhalation, the diaphragm relaxes upwards, takes dome shape, allows the ribs to drop down and in with flattened belly that causes chest cavity to contract back to normal state. This contraction in thoracic volume causes increase in the pressure of carbon dioxide rich air (in the alveoli) in the chest cavity leading to its expulsion to the atmosphere through the respiratory tract (due to pressure differential with the atmospheric air).

The acts of breathing during inhalation and exhalation as mentioned above are pictorially illustrated in figure no. 5.

13. BREATHING PARAMETERS

The volume of air that a person breathes in and out under normal circumstances is called tidal volume (TV). Tidal Volume (TV) basically represents the volume of air that is inhaled or exhaled under normal circumstances when no extra pressure is applied either during inhalation or during exhalation. It is around 500 milliliter for adults both for men as well as for women (refer table no. 2).

When a person consciously inhales air with application of force, he draws more air from the atmosphere than he does in normal inhalation. Likewise, when a person exhales with application of force, he exhales more air than he does in normal exhalation.

With application of force, the additional air that a person can inhale above the normal inspirational volume i.e. tidal volume, is known as **inspiratory reserve volume (IRV)**. It is around 3.0 litres for adult men and 1.9 litres for adult women (refer table no. 2). Likewise, the additional air that can be forcibly exhaled by a person after the expiration of normal tidal volume is known as **expiratory reserve volume (ERV)**, which is around 1.1 litre for adult men and 0.7 litre for adult women (refer table no. 2).

During exhalation, even if a person forcibly breathes out as much as he possibly can, he still can not push out and eliminate all of the air from the respiratory tract. The amount of air which still remains in the chest cavity even after forced exhalation is called residual volume. **Residual volume (RV)** therefore can be described as the volume of air which still remains in the lungs after the expiratory reserve volume is exhaled. It is around 1.2 litre for adult men and 1.1 litre for adult women (refer table no. 2). It is to be noted here that the existence of a total vacuum in the respiratory tract is undesired as it may cause the 'tract' to buckle. The various breathing parameters discussed above are tabled in table no. 2 below.

PARAMETERS	AVERAGE VALUES IN LITRES	
	ADULT MEN	ADULT WOMEN
Tidal volume..... .... (TV)	0.5	0.5
Inspiratory reserve volume ....(IVR)	3.0	1.9
Expiratory reserve volume ....(ERV)	1.1	0.7
Residual volume............... (RV)	1.2	1.1

Table no. 2

14. MAXIMUM BREATHING POTENTIAL

The maximum amount of air a person can expel after maximum inhalation is called his vital capacity (VC). Vital Capacity (VC) is the sum total of tidal volume (TV), the inspiratory reserve volume (IRV) and expiratory reserve volume (ERV).

VC= TV +IRV + ERV.

When the air that always remains in the respiratory system i.e. the residual volume (RV) is added with the amount of air that a person can ever inhale i.e. his vital capacity (VC), then the total amount is referred to as total lung capacity (TLC). So, total lung capacity (TLC) is the sum total of vital capacity (VC) and residual volume (RV)

TLC = VC + RV = TV + IRV + ERV + RV.

The maximum potential of inhalation is the sum total of tidal volume (TV) and the inspiratory reserve volume (IRV). This is known as inspiratory capacity (IC).

IC = TV + IRV.

It has been mentioned earlier that normally a person exhales only the tidal volume of air (TV) and the additional amount of air that can be exhaled through application of force is known as expiratory reserve volume (ERV). It has further been mentioned that the amount of air that remains inside even after forced exhalation is known as reserve volume. The sum total of the additional air that can be exhaled with application of force i.e. expiratory reserve volume (ERV) and the volume that remains in the respiratory tract even after forced exhalation i.e. reserve volume (RV) is called the functional residual capacity (FRC).

FRC = RV + ERV

Vital capacity (VC), inspiratory capacity (IC), functional residual capacity (FRC) and total lung capacity (TLC) of average adult men and women are tabled in table no. 3.

PARAMETERS	AVERAGE VALUE IN LITRES	
	ADULT MEN	ADULT WOMEN
Vital Capacity VC = TV +IRV + ERV	4.6	3.1
Inspiratory Capacity IC = VC + IRV	3.5	2.4
Functional Residual Capacity FRC = RV + ERV	2.3	1.8
Total Lung Capacity TLC = VC + RV = TV + IRV + ERV + RV	5.8	4.2

Table no. 3

Along with the capacity of breathing, it is important for a person to understand and follow the rhythm and the different types of breathing.

15. IDENTIFICATION OF THE BREATHING PATTERN

To follow the rhythms of breathing, a person has to be conversant with the basic types of breathing. It is a fact of life that even though every individual is constantly inhaling and exhaling, most of them are unaware of the type of breathing they adapt and the phenomenal impact that the breathing has on their well being. It is said that breathing is the way of life; the way a person breathes, is the way he lives.

To identify the breathing pattern, a person has to concentrate on each specific steps of his natural breathing without exercising control in any way. To start with, he has to relax and lie down flat on his back with the left hand on the chest and right hand on the navel area and follow with full attention the flowing of breathe

1. in and out of the nose/mouth,
2. in and out at the back of the mouth above the throat,

3. through the throat area up and down,
4. in and out of the trachea through the bronchioles into the alveoli in the lungs (discussed in section 06, 07,08 & 09). During this stage, the expansion and relaxation of the chest and downward and upward movement of the abdomen is to be felt through the rising and falling of the left and right hand respectively.

The above exercise is continued for a number of breathing cycles. If a person feels with his left hand that the chest expands and contracts with each breath while the abdominal area does not, then he is said to be on chest breathing or thoracic breathing. If on the other hand the right hand feels that the abdomen moves up and down with each breath with little movement of the chest, then the person is said to be on abdomen breathing or diaphragmatic breathing.

Other than chest breathing and abdominal breathing, there are other types of breathing too. The details of the different types of breathings clubbed in groups are discussed in the subsequent section.

16. DIFFFERENT BREATHING PRACTICES

All types of breathing practices can broadly be clubbed into three groups – chest breathing, abdominal breathing and clavicular breathing. There is also another type of breathing practice called paradoxical breathing. Paradoxical breathing is very uncommon; a person generally resorts to this type of breathing under various types of medical problems.

Chest breathing or thoracic breathing: Chest breathing uses chest muscles to inflate the lungs by pulling on the rib cage. In chest breathing, the chest expands and contracts with each breath while the abdominal area does not. During conscious chest breathing,

1. while inhaling, a person discontinues the use of diaphragm and starts to inhale by slowly expanding the ribcage and eventually expands it as much as possible. He feels the movement of the individual ribs outwards and upwards with

the awareness that this expansion allows the air to be drawn into the lungs,

2. while exhaling, the person feels the relaxation of the chest muscles along with the feelings of ribcage contraction. He also feels the air forcing out of the lungs.

The entire cycle of chest breathing is performed through expansion and contraction of the chest without making use of the diaphragm. In general, chest breathing uses only a small portion of the lungs and delivers relatively minimal amount of oxygen to the bloodstream. It is often associated with the sensation of 'feeling out of breath'. Through chest breathing, a person attempts to take in oxygen quickly despite the low air volume from each breath. It-

1. is useful during vigorous exercise but is quite inappropriate for ordinary, everyday activity,
2. is predominant when an individual is aroused by external or internal challenges or danger. It is also associated with other symptoms of arousal like tension and anxiety.

With 'chest breathing', the breath is generally shallow, jerky and unsteady, resulting in unsteadiness of the mind and emotions. Until chest breathing is replaced by deep, even and steady diaphragmatic breathing, all efforts to relax the body, nerves and mind will be ineffective.

Abdominal or stomach or diaphragmatic or belly breathing: Abdominal breathing also known as stomach breathing or diaphragmatic breathing or belly breathing refers to the breathing practice that uses the entire lung capacity. During inhalation, the diaphragm contracts and the dome flattens and moves downward into the abdominal cavity. This movement increases the thoracic cavity; the increase being directly proportional to the amount of the 'movement' of reference. The diaphragm contraction also induces the lower ribs to move upward and forward, which further increases the thoracic volume. In the abdominal breathing, the chest expands very little if at all, while the abdominal area expands significantly.

Abdominal breathing is slow and deep, takes longer to inhale and exhale and delivers a significantly larger amount of oxygen to the bloodstream. The larger amount of air intake also allows exhalation of larger amount of carbon dioxide, eliminating it from the body at a faster rate. With abdominal breathing, a person generally feels calm and composed. It is the most important tool available for stress management. It promotes a natural, even movement of breath which both strengthens the nervous system and relaxes the body. It is the most efficient method of breathing, using minimum effort for maximum oxygen. Abdominal breathing increases endurance by providing much more oxygen to the bloodstream, allowing the body to generate more energy.

Clavicular breathing: Clavicular breathing is significant when maximum air is needed. It is the extended stage of ribcage expansion after the thoracic inhalation is completed. The name is so derived from the two clavicles or collar bones which are pulled up slightly at the end of maximum inhalation. It comes into play when the body's need for oxygen is very acute. This type of breathing is generally done by patients with asthma or chronic bronchitis.

Paradoxical breathing: Paradoxical breathing describes an abnormal chest movement, with the chest moving inward during inhalation rather than outward. This abnormal movement impairs the ability to effectively inhale, limiting the amount of oxygen a person can take in. Blood oxygen levels drop and carbon dioxide levels increase, because this metabolic byproduct cannot be exhaled adequately. Various types of medical problems can lead to paradoxical breathing by disrupting different aspects of normal breathing mechanism. For example, traumatic injury to the thorax, in which several ribs are fractured in two or more places and are no longer attached by bony cartilage to the rest of the rib cage often lead to paradoxical breathing. Patients with chronic air passageway obstruction also experience paradoxical breathing.

17. ADVANTAFE OF ABDOMINAL BREATHING

Free, long and rhythmic diaphragmatic breathing is the key to the enhancement of physical and emotional well being. The diaphragm is a large muscle that divides the trunk of the body into two chambers. The upper chamber houses the heart and lungs, and the lower chamber houses the digestive organs stomach, liver, intestines, etc. Unlike other muscles which are either controlled voluntarily through the central nervous system or involuntarily through the autonomic nervous system (refer section 47 of part three), the diaphragm muscle is unique in the sense that it functions under both voluntary and involuntary control. As mentioned in section 15 above, it is the most efficient method of breathing which uses minimum effort for maximum oxygen and is the most important tool available for stress management.

Diaphragmatic breathing is the most natural way the new born babies breathe. If the breathing of babies is observed, it will be seen that they fully use their diaphragm/belly with each breath. They are able to do so because their mind is totally free from any kind of thoughts. They have no past to remember, no future to plan or any worry to bother about. To them every breath is simply a process of receiving from the universe and giving back to it. Because they exist only on 'now', they continue to breathe freely and effortlessly and experience peace, joy and connectedness with all the surroundings.

As babies grow into adults, they start developing different postures, anxious thinking, tension and pressures arising out of external influences. They start bothering about what is right and what is wrong and also become conscious about what others are thinking of them. Arising out of their proximity to the surrounding environments, wittingly as well as unwittingly, they slowly develop their own perceptions from their experiences. In order to be good and acceptable to the environment, they often have cross thoughts within. This causes tightening of different muscles in their body which adversely affect their breathing pattern. Their mind starts racing with thoughts, they lose the freedom, joy and expansiveness that they were enjoying as babies and as a result they make departure from the normal abdominal breathing of their baby days. They resort to breathing by lifting their chest. Since the chest muscles are not designed to continually inflate and deflate the lungs, they fatigue when called upon to do so. It therefore becomes impossible for the adults to properly inflate the lungs by using the chest muscles. The tissues in the process get chronically deprived of oxygen—the most important "nutrient" the body needs for good health.

To revert back to natural abdominal breathing of the baby days, the grown up adults have to let go of the patterns of racing thoughts embracing worries, anxieties and tensions by consciously calming the mind from time to time. Through application of numbers of breathing practices

1. a buzzing mind can be brought to rest,
2. stress and anxiety can be lowered with increase in vitality,
3. energy can be made to soar when a person feels low on it,
4. concentration can be improved with restoration of balance and calmness of mind by bringing into harmony the left and right hemispheres of the brain which correlate to the logical and emotional sides of human personality.

A teacher of proven credential can guide and help a person to adapt specific breathing practices to tide over different circumstances and situations to lead a fruitful and meaningful life. For general awareness, benefits of application of some of the proven breathing practices are discussed in section 51 of part three.

18. BREATH AND EMOTION

Emotions are strong feelings of a person arising out of his circumstances, moods or his relationships with others. They broadly are classified into two categories, namely love based emotion like joy, happiness, caring, trust, compassion, truth, contentment, satisfaction etc., and fear based emotion like anxiety, anger, control, sadness, depression, inadequacy, confusion, hurt, lonely, guilt, shame etc. Though emotions generally are identified as either negative or positive, they basically are nothing but raw energies. What a person does with them eventually determine whether they bring him negative or positive consequences. For example,

1. when a person simply succumbs to anger, he expends energy in a negative way, but if he channelizes anger and converts it into inspiration or challenge to achieve something, it becomes a positive energy.
2. when fear causes worries and anxieties, energy is expended in a negative way, but if the causes of fear are identified and a person prepares, acts and updates himself to neutralize its possible negative impact, it becomes a positive energy. Napoleon was once asked if he feared bad luck. He replied in affirmative and said that he always believed he would have it, and he planned and prepared accordingly.

Emotions need to be given full expressions. Suppression of the causes of emotion adversely affects a person physically as well as mentally, like

1. anger weakens the liver,
2. grief weakens the lungs,
3. worry weakens the stomach,
4. stress weakens heart and brain,
5. fear weakens the kidney, so on and so forth.

That emotions are directly linked to rhythms and patterns of breathing (refer section 19 of part one) generally goes unnoticed to a person even though he himself experiences and sees others experiencing the same every day. There are number of breathing practices (refer section 51 of part three) through which emotional states can immediately be addressed to and the mind be helped to release pent up or repressed emotion and return back to normalcy. Subsequently however, the root cause of the emotion has to be identified and an appropriate methodology has to be developed to deal with and neutralize the possible long stretch adverse affects of the emotion.

19. INFLUENCE OF BREATH ON EMOTION

The rhythm of the breath is one of the most obvious physical indications of a person's emotional and mental state. It is relevant to quote Sri Sri Ravi Shankar in this context. While addressing a conference, he once said, "Our breath is linked to our emotions. For every emotion, there is a particular rhythm in the breath. So, when you directly cannot harness your emotion, with the help of breath you can do it. If you are in a theater, you know that a director would ask you to breathe faster when you have to show anger. If you have to show serene scene, the director would tell you to breathe softer and slower. If we understand the rhythm of our breath, we are able to have a say over our mind."

Each basic emotional state whether it is love based or fear based has a breathing pattern associated with it. For example,

1. panic is associated with short, fast, shallow breaths,
2. anger is associated with long and forced breaths,
3. calmness is associated with slow and steady breaths,
4. happiness is associated with long inhalations and long exhalations and so forth.

When a person is angry, fearful, or anxious, he over-breathes or in common parlance, 'huffs and puffs'. In case of sadness, suspense, conflict or depression, a person under-breathes i.e. he 'holds his breath'.

Sri Sri Ravi Shankar further said, "The mind is like a kite, flying here and there, and the breath is like the string of the kite, generally bringing the mind back into the present moment. The breath brings the mind, which is all over the place, back to its source, a natural state of peacefulness and joy." Bringing the mind under control through proper application of breath therefore is of paramount importance.

For centuries, expert practitioners employed specific breathing techniques to calm down the mind and address emotions under different circumstances. For example, when a person feels sluggish, application of bhastrika pranayam gives him immediate surge of energy and invigorates the mind; when a person feels angry, irritated or frustrated, application of ujjayi breathing immediately soothes and settles his mind, so on and so forth.

Learning to consciously and deliberately regulate the breath is a key to mastery over both emotions and the mind. While the negative emotions cause over breathing, under breathing and irregular breathing, the positive emotions cause breathing to be deeper, slower, easier and effortless. By the above functional relationship, when a person restores his breathing to a deeper, smooth and rhythmical pattern, he reduces the influence of negative emotions and acquires a peaceful and relaxing mental state. To manage emotional states through breathing, a person needs to practice different breathing techniques (some of them are discussed in section 51 of part three) to influence emotions not just whenever he is in the strong grip of them, but daily, as a routine, much like brushing of his teeth.

20. ASANA & CHANTING OF MANTRAS

Along with air intake and carbon dioxide elimination, breathing is also associated with intake of subtle prana into the body. Prana, a source of multifarious energy (discussed in details in part two and part three) is drawn from universal prana and is distributed to different parts of the body through breath.

Asana has profound influence in uninterrupted distribution of prana in the mind and body complex. While a posture is any particular position of the body, an asana is defined as the state of being in which a person can remain physically and mentally steady, calm and comfortable for a long period. Apart from sitting, modern usage of asana includes lying on the back, standing on the head and a variety of other positions. In the Yoga Sutras, Patanjali suggests asanas as 'sthiram sukham asanam' meaning, that position which is comfortable and steady. In reality, asanas are considered to be the specific body positions which open the pranic energy channels (refer nadis in section 32 of part two) and psychic centres (refer section 36 of part two) for the free flow of prana in the body with the breath. Asanas in which various breathing exercises (yogic) are performed are known as yogasana. Specific breathing practices in identified postures produce different energetic, mental, emotional and physical effects.

Sounds also have different effects on human psyche like

1. soft sound of wind rusting through, soothes the nerves,
2. musical notes of running stream enchants the heart,
3. thunder cause scare and fear, so on and so forth.

The sacred utterances/ chanting of mantras provide mankind with the power to get transformed from the ordinary to the higher level of consciousness, especially during performing spiritual breathing practices.

PART TWO

BREATH & PRANA

It is interesting to quote Indian poet Kabir in the context of flow of prana in the human body. He once said, "God is a breath within the breath". His statement had wide implications; what he meant was that beyond the physical components of breath (oxygen, carbon dioxide etc.), within it, there is prana, a divine presence. This prana is derived from the divine source of universal prana. It is an energy which commences within the human being as soon as a person is conceived in the mother's womb. As the body formation takes place and the person starts breathing, he goes on drawing more of prana from the universal prana with his breath on a regular basis.

Prana keeps human life functioning and is the prime mover of all the activities starting from gross physical movement to minute biochemical processes in the human body. It is prana which is responsible even for the act of human breathing. The moment flow of prana in the body stops, a person's breathing will also stop automatically. A breathing body is alive, but a breathless body becomes a 'dead body'. Prana flows in human body as different vayus. Each vayu has specific functions in identified parts of the body. Through the process of breathing, prana as vayus are circulated throughout the mind, body complex via innumerable numbers of subtle nadis. These nadis are connected to numbers of subtle chakras at different locations of the body. Chakras form the distributing centres for prana vayus within the body. Through specific breathing exercises, the flow of prana vayus can be regulated within the body to bring about improvement in the physical and mental life.

21. PRANA, THE VITAL FORCE

From time immemorial, all the wise people of this planet regardless of the traditions they belonged/belong to attested/attest to the fact that there exists a fundamental divine energy in the universe that

1. transcends the time and space,
2. impregnates all the things and beings in this universe,
3. influences the life and health of living beings.

This fundamental and divine energy is air borne and is known as universal energy or vital energy or prana shakti or universal prana or simply as prana. Although closely related to the air mankind breathes in, it is more subtle (refer section 41 of part three) than air or oxygen. Prana is all pervading. Everything on earth, including the human being is born through prana and lives by it. As per yogic philosophy prana commences within the human being as soon as a person is conceived in the mother's womb. As the body formation takes place and a person starts the process of breathing, he goes on drawing more and more of prana from the universal prana on a regular basis.

Prana is similar to electricity in that it is not physically seen but supplies an invisible current and keeps life flowing and functioning. It is the prime mover of all the activities starting from gross physical movement to minute biochemical processes in the human body. Prana is responsible even for the act of breathing. The moment flow of prana in the body stops, a person's breathing stops automatically. A breathing body is alive, but a breathless body becomes a 'dead body'.

Prana is circulated throughout the mind - body complex via innumerable numbers of subtle nadis (refer section 32 of part two) through breath. These nadis are connected to numbers of subtle chakras (discussed in details in section 36 of part two) at different locations of the body. Chakras form the distributing centres of prana within the body. Prana flows to different parts of the body as vayus. Effects of the flow of prana in the body are visible in the physical plane as motion and action and in the mental plane as thought.

22. PRANA IS INDESTRUCTIBLE

When it enters human body, prana is clean and pure, but gets contaminated as it flows through the body. How it departs the body depends upon an individual's life style, food habits, inner qualities, feelings, environment etc. The quality of the prana that radiates from people impacts on both the surrounding environment and the individuals themselves.

Emotional distress affects the flow of prana. The more a person feels disheartened or depressed, the weaker is the flow of prana; this leaves him susceptible to illness, and his aging process also occurs more rapidly. On the other hand, a balanced and content person radiates vitality, and his strength reaches out to touch fellow human beings. A person therefore, should always adapt specific breathing practices to cleanse the passageways of prana and ensure its uninterrupted free flow.

Total amount of universal prana is fixed and is indestructible. It however changes form from energy to matter and again from matter to energy. It also changes from one form of energy into another form of energy. Everything in this universe is made up of matter and energy. Matter is anything that occupies space, has mass and contains energy. Energy on the other hand has no mass, occupies no space but is capable of moving matters. When a being or a material substance reaches the end of its cycle life or independent existence, the energy that had sustained it so far is re-absorbed into the universal prana as non-differentiated universal prana.

23. PRANA IS MULTIFARIOUS ENERGY

It is a common knowledge that water is a potential source of multifarious energies. When water from a river is held in a dam, the river turns into a lake. Here the potential energy of the river water gets held back from flowing. But when the river water is made to flow and channeled towards a power generating plant, it becomes an active energy of motion called kinetic energy. In the power plant, when the flowing water hits the blades of the turbines, the water energy is converted into rotational mechanical energy. This mechanical energy is transferred from the turbine through a shaft to the generator which converts the mechanical energy into electrical energy via transformer; it is then transferred to different destinations centres from where the electricity is utilized for various purposes. Like water, prana too is a source of multifarious energy. In the human body prana functions in the form of different energies like

1. physical energy (energy that one manipulates daily),
2. mental energy (when the mind gathers information),
3. intellectual energy (when information is analyzed & filtered),
4. electrical energy (when the brain emanates oscillating electrical voltage of the order in few millionths of a volt).
5. spiritual energy when it flows though sushumna (refer section 52 of part three), so on and so forth.

24. PRANA & SPIRITUAL CONSCIOUNESS

Prana, the primal source of all forms of energies manifests itself in various frequencies. A person's level of consciousness determines the frequencies of prana he is capable of receiving from the universal prana.

No two individual minds and bodies are alike; accordingly their need for prana is different; it is therefore not possible to quantify in absolute terms the amount of prana an individual needs. A person can develop the capacity to store additional amount of prana through the practice of 'pranayama' (refer section 51 of part three).

Every person carries certain amount of prana in the body; while a substantial portion of it is utilized in the course of his day to day activities throughout his life, part of it lies dormant at the base of the spine which he can utilize towards his quest for spiritual consciousness. The journey from the physical level to spiritual realm requires vast quantity of energy. This energy can be supplied by the 'dormant' prana when activated. Through wide range of specific breathing practices, a person can awaken the dormant and static prana from her slumber, lead her up through the sushumna (refer section 49 of part three) , pass all the chakras (refer section 36 of part two) and meet the shiva shakti at the shahasrara to attain spiritual consciousness (refer section 55 of part three).

It must however be known that in order to achieve spiritual consciousness, resorting only to breathing techniques is not enough; a person has to direct his whole life towards everything good. The person must be free from hatred, greed, anger, envy, jealousy, passion and dependency; he must live in love, harmony and understanding with the environment. When the specific breathing practices and the positive way of life (as mentioned above) merge with each other, a person makes progress in his spiritual journey.

25. SOURCES OF PRANA

The function of human body is much like a transformer, receiving energy from the universal flow of prana and distributing that energy and then eliminating it. Apart from the prana that commences within the human body as soon as a person in born as mentioned in section 21 of part two, the other sources from which prana enters into the human body are

1. solar prana,
2. air prana,
3. earth prana,
4. food including water.

Solar prana: Solar prana is the energy drawn from the sun. Sun is the source of powerful heat, light and energy.

Air prana: Air prana is the energy drawn from the atmosphere through the process of inhalation. With specific practices of slow and rhythmic breathing, absorption of air prana can be enhanced. Maximum intake of energy to the human body is through air prana.

Earth prana: Earth prana or ground prana is the energy drawn from the ground through soles of the feet.

Trees and plants absorb prana from sun, air, and earth and exude a lot of excess prana. Sick or physically exhausted people are often asked to rest underneath trees basically to reap the benefit of this excess prana.

Food and water: Drinking sun exposed water transfers solar prana to the human body. All foods grown on earth derive energy from the earth prana, even the foods soaked under sun rays derive solar prana. Through eating of these foods, prana gets transferred to the human body.

26. ABSORPTION & EXIT OF PRANA

Solar prana is absorbed mostly from the sun rays through 'exposure', skin being the absorption medium. Solar prana also enters the body while drinking sun soaked water, mouth being the absorption medium.

Air prana is absorbed during inhalation. Entry of air prana is mostly through the nasal cavity, though it can also be absorbed through the mouth.

Earth prana is absorbed through feet; connecting directly with the earth by walking barefoot outdoors best facilitates this unconscious process.

When food is taken, its unprocessed energy derived from earth prana and solar prana get transferred to the human body, the medium of absorption being the mouth.

Extensive research conducted reveals that there are nine openings (eyes 2, ears 2, nostrils 2, mouth 1, sex organ 1, anus 1) and the skin through which prana enters and the spent energy leaves the human body.

In general, maximum percentage of energy (around 65 %) enters human body through the nostrils (inhalation being the medium) followed by around 30 % through the mouth (intake of food and water and inhalation in some cases). On an average 50 % of the spent energy leaving the body finds exit through nostrils (as carbon dioxide during exhalation) followed by around 43 % through skin as sweat etc.

27. UTILISATION OF PRANA

Extensive research works reveal that 70 % of the prana is utilized in carrying out various activities on regular basis (as mentioned underneath) while 30 % remains dormant in the form of kundalini shakti which is utilized during spiritual growth.

Out of the 70 % of the prana utilized on regular basis, 20 % is used by the physical body (12 % for voluntary actions and 8 % for involuntary actions) and 50 % is used by the subtle body. Breakup of the 50 % of the energy expended on the subtle body (refer section 41 of part three) is mentioned underneath.

1. Conscious mind - 5 %. Conscious mind creates ideas, desires, dreams, feels, remembers, imagines, produces thoughts through the five human senses (refer section 58 of part three).
2. Sub conscious mind - 23 % (Give and take centre 3 %, like and dislike centre 4 %, desire centre 8 %, temperamental centre 8 %). Subconscious mind stores thoughts that have been funneled repeatedly by the conscious mind. These thoughts get ingrained in the subconscious system as retrievable memories which on stimulation function in auto mode. The subconscious mind stores these thoughts in a systematic manner as different cabinets like
   i. give and take centre that maintains all types of 'give and take' accounts. It often tries to settle scores with others whenever and wherever opportunity permits,

ii. likes and dislikes centre that stores impressions on likes and dislikes and on stimulation sends impulses back to the conscious mind,
iii. desire centre that stores all desires and instincts,
iv. temperamental centre that stores the temperamental characteristics of individuals.

3. Intellect - 15 % (interpretation centre 7.5 % and intellect centre 7.5 %). Intellect rationalizes, discerns, chooses, compares, decides, understands, analyses, identifies and evaluates.
4. Ego – 7 %. Ego is the focus of conscious attention.

Since vast quantity of prana is needed to raise the energy from physical to the spiritual realms, a person desirous of attaining spiritual consciousness, has to exercise conscious control on his voluntary physical and mental activities like eating of food, sexual behavior, emotion, thought, imagination etc. and also store prana through the practice of pranayama. As far as intake of food is concerned, the amount, the type, the timing and the manner of eating play an important role. Irregularities in life style arising out of dietary indiscretions and stress cause obstruction in the flow of prana in specific part of the body leading to devitalization of related organs and limbs. It can also lead to metabolic dysfunction.

28. PRANA FUNCTIONS AS DIFFERENT VAYUS

Prana functions in the human body as vayus (wind) and is carried to different parts of the body with the breath. It is said that it gets divided into 49 vayus and flows through subtle channels (refer section 32 of part two) throughout the mind – body complex. Based on major regulatory and vital activities performed by them, five prana vayus and five sub prana vayus are identified to play very important roles. The flow channels of the different vayus can be cleansed through application of specific breathing practices under the guidance of a teacher of proven credentials.

The five important vayus are prana vayu, apana vayu, samana vayu, udana vayu and vyana vayu. Collectively these five vayus are known as pancha pranas or pancha bhutas. Five important sub prana vayus are naga vayu, korma vayu, devdatta vayu, krikala vayu and dhananjaya vayu.

Prana vayu operates in the upper part of the body and is responsible for the activity of inhalation. Apana vayu stabilizes the lower part of the body and is responsible for the activities of urination, excretion, ejaculation, child birth etc. Vyana vayu controls the fluid movements and is responsible for the activities of voluntary and involuntary movements within and outside the body. Samana vayu plays between the navel and the rib cage that balances prana vayu and apana vayu and is responsible for the activities of stomach and intestines. Udana vayu ascends from the collar bones and passes through the neck, throat and head. It is responsible for the activities of exhalation and speech.

29. VAYUS ARE INTERLINKED

The pancha pranas representing the five main important vayus are not exactly the separate manifestations of prana. They represent different functions of the prana as vayus in the human body. Though they function together in unison, each one of these vayus moves in specific directions and specific regions of the human body, it activates specific physiological and bodily processes as mentioned below. The flow of these vayus can be controlled by appropriate breathing techniques. It is always advisable that these techniques of breathing are learned under the guidance of a Guru or teacher of proven credentials.

All the five important vayus are intimately linked to each other. One can enjoy health and well-being only if all these five vayus are balanced and work in harmony. While the prana vayu and udana vayu move upwards and are known as energy of collection and assimilation, the apana vayu moves downwards and is known as energy of elimination. Samana vayu represents the energy of contraction while vyana vayu is called the energy of expansion. Flow patterns of the pancha pranas, their individual characteristics and what happens when there is blockage in the channels of their flow are summarized in table no. 4.

DIFFERENT PRANA VAYUS	FLOW PATTERN	FUNCTIONAL LOCATION	FUNCTIONAL ACTIVITY	BLOCKAGES IN FLOW AFFECTS
Prana vayu	Inward moving	Heart, chest, lungs	Respiration, sensory perception.	Heart, Lungs and digestive system
Apana vayu	Descending	Below the navel	Elimination, reproduction and child birth.	Menstrual cycle, sexual function etc. and bowel movements
Samana vayu	Equalizing	Navel	Digestion, metabolism and homeo-stasis.	Digestive system.
Vyana vayu	All pervasive	Pervades entire body including perepheral nervous sys-tem	Movements and circula-tions.	Peripheral circulation causing numbness in different parts of the body
Udana vayu	Ascending	Throat, Upper chest and Head.	Thought, speech, ner-vous system	Cognition, communica-tion.

Table no. 4

30. DESCRIPTION OF PANCHA PRANAS

Details of the characteristics and functions of the pancha prana vayus are mentioned underneath.

PRANA VAYU

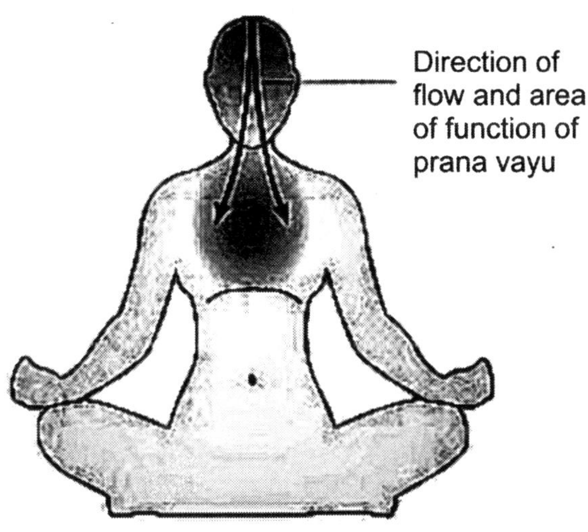

Figure no. 6

Prana vayu moves inward and governs the movement of energy from the head down to the navel area which is the pranic centre of the physical body. Its main area of function covers the thoracic region, face, ears, nose, tongue and the brain. Direction of flow of prana vayu and its area of function is shown in figure no. 6.

Prana vayu is responsible for the proper functioning of the respiratory system and the vital organs, particularly the heart. Intake of energy through inhalation of air, eating of food, drinking of water, reception of sensory impressions and ideas etc. are all regulated by prana vayu. It maintains body temperature with respect to the prevailing environment and is the fundamental energy in the body; it directs and feeds into the other four important vayus. Reduction in the balance of prana vayu leads to depression and lethargy. Prana vayu is the source of power for the anahata chakra (chakras have been discussed in detail at section 36 of part two).

APANA VAYU

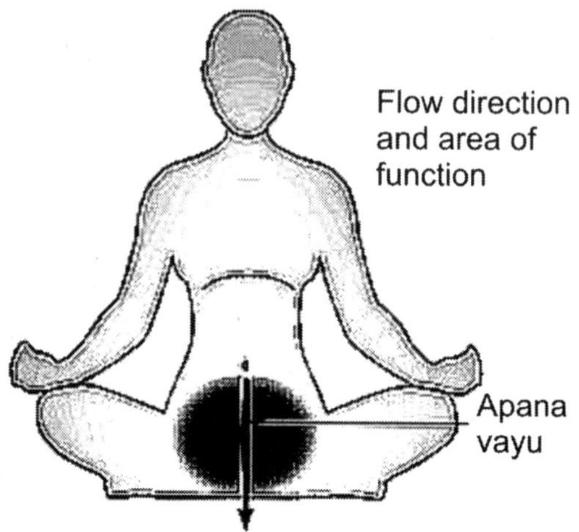

Figure no. 7

Apana vayu flows downwards and outwards and governs the movement of energy from the navel down to the floor of the pelvis. Its energy nourishes the organs of digestion, reproduction and elimination. Direction of flow of apana vayu and its area of function is shown in figure no. 7.

Apana vayu regulates

1. the elimination of the stool and the urine,
2. expelling of semen, menstrual fluid etc.,
3. elimination of carbon dioxide through the breath.

On the subtle level, apana vayu eliminates not only physical wastes but also anything undesirable or derogatory to good health. It supports the immune system and helps keep the mind free of destructive forces. Disturbance in the flow of apana vayu leads to diseases in lower abdomen embracing intestines, kidneys, urinary tract etc. Apana vayu is the source of power for the mooladhara chakra.

SAMANA VAYU

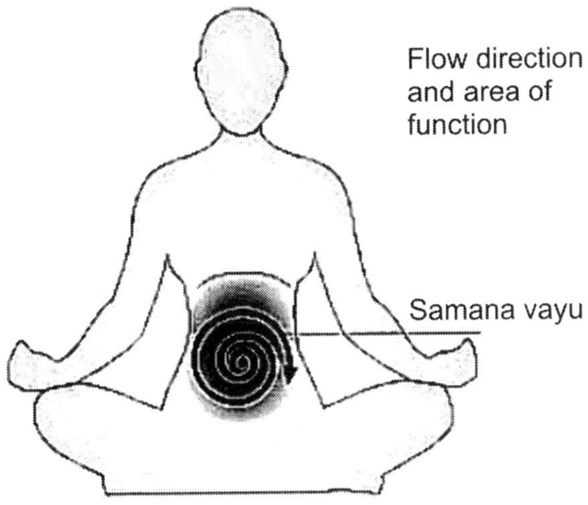

Figure no. 8

Samana vayu rules between the navel and the rib cage and plays the role of balancing act between the two opposing forces of prana vayu and the apana vayu. Direction of flow of samana vayu and its area of function is shown in figure no. 8.

Samana vayu moves from the periphery to the centre and participates in the metabolic activities involved in digestion. It works in the gastrointestinal tract and the lungs. From the incoming substances drawn in by the prana vayu, it digests energy and assimilates sensory impressions and ideas. It separates the portions of the digested food from waste products and assists in their elimination. Imbalance in samana vayu leads to improper function of the digestive organs as well as disruption in mental ability which assimilates ideas and impressions. Samana vayu is the source of power for the manipura chakra.

UDANA VAYU

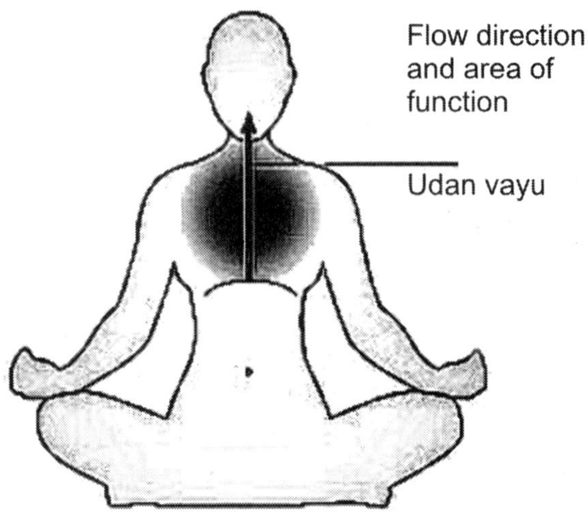

Figure no. 9

Udana vayu, also known as 'ascending air' is the energy that ascends from the collar bones and passes through the neck, throat and head on inhalation it circulates throughout the head and the sense organs like ears, nose, eyes, mouth etc. on exhalation. Direction of flow of udana vayu and its area of function is shown in figure no. 9. Udana vayu makes a person feel confident, assertive and helps him to express himself articulately. When udana vayu is in imbalance, one finds it difficult to communicate properly; conversations become inappropriate with either loss of words or too many words. The energy of udana vayu helps a person to raise the bar in order to achieve higher aspirations; it also enhances his power of intuition. It is the energy which helps in self transformation and spiritual growth.

Udana vayu is activated by samana vayu which itself is activated by the balance of prana vayu and apana vayu. When prana vayu and apana vayu flows freely, udana vayu functions optimally. On death of a person, the udana vayu draws the soul up and out of the body. Udana vayu is the source of power for the vishudhi chakra.

VYANA VAYU

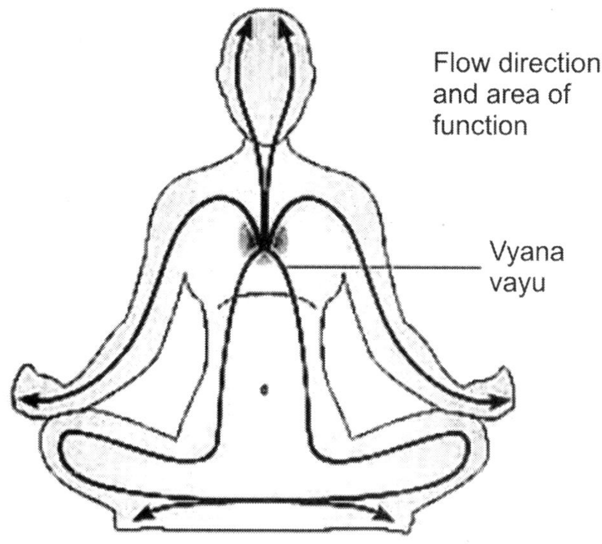

Figure no. 10

Vyana vayu is the outward moving energy from the heart and the lungs that flows towards the periphery throughout the human body. Direction of flow of vyana vayu and its area of function is shown in figure no. 10. It governs all the circulatory channels and moves the food, water and oxygen throughout the body. It keeps human emotions and thoughts circulating in the mind and acts as reserve energy for other primary important vayus that require an extra boost to carry out their functions. It controls the muscular system and movements from the core to the periphery and is responsible for voluntary as well as involuntary relaxation and concentration of all muscles. Vyana vayu is the source of power for the swadhisthana chakra.

31. DESCRIPTION OF FIVE IMPORTANT SUB PRANA VAYUS

The five important sub prana vayus are naga vayu, korma vayu, devdatta vayu, krikala vayu and dhananjaya vayu. While naga vayu controls burping, kurma vayu performs the function of opening and closing of the eyes, krikala vayu induces hunger and thirst, devadatta vayu does yawning and dhananjaya vayu causes decomposition of the body after death.

Naga vayu is responsible for controlling 'burping' (noisy expulsion of wind from the stomach through mouth) and helps in the removal of blockages in the flow of prana vayu and apana vayu and prevents gas formation in the digestive system. It also helps in triggering of the vomit reflex due to indigestion and dissolves blockages in the flow of samana vayu. Suppression of 'burping' may lead to cardiac disorder.

Koorma vayu is responsible for controlling contracting movements e.g. blinking (shutting and opening of eyes quickly). Its areas of functions are eyes. Basically it controls the opening and closing of the eye lids. The energy of the korma vayu is active when a person is awake and is revitalized when he goes to sleep. Its natural instinct is to protect the eyes from the penetration of dust and foreign bodies etc. In a state of imbalance it can cause uncontrolled blinking and twitching of the eyelids. The practice of trataka provides balance and strength to korma vayu, as does the chanting of OM, placing of warm palms over the eyes and asanas where the head is bent forward.

Trataka is the practice of fixed staring at some external object. This fixed gazing is a method which enables a person to concentrate on a single point such as a small object, black dot or candle flame etc. It helps in the purification of eyes, strengthening of the eye muscles, and leads to improvement in vision, memory and concentration of the mind in preparation for stimulating the ajna chakra.

Devdatta vayu is responsible for controlling of 'yawning' (deep breathing with mouth open to expel gas and reduce tiredness after eating). Its function is similar to that of samana vayu. Certain foods such as grains, onions and garlic cause fatigue. Many people only eat vegetables and some milk products in order to sustain their level of vitality and thereby reduce lethargy.

Krikala vayu is responsible for controlling hunger, thirst, sneezing and coughing. Sneezing (sudden expulsion of air from the nose and mouth due to irritation in the nostrils) in particular helps in clearing blockages in the respiratory tract; it also releases energy blockages in the head and neck area. Suppression of sneeze adversely affects the cervical spine. Weak sneeze indicate weak vitality.

Dhananjaya vayu influences the whole body and in particular the muscles of the heart by opening and closing the heart valves. It governs the decomposition of the body and persists for sometime even after one's death.

Prana vayus and sub prana vayus vayus flow through identified channels and are distributed throughout the entire mind body complex via energy centres. These energy channels are known as nadis and the distributing energy centres are known as chakras.

32. THE NADIS

Nadis are the passageways through which the fundamental energy of life - prana is transmitted throughout the human body. Unlike normal nadis of the physical body, the nadis carrying prana do not have physical manifestations; they are subtle (refer section 41 of part three). While the gross nadis of the physical body comprises of blood vessels, arteries, veins etc., the subtle nadis are imperceptible conduits of prana. They cannot be physically seen with naked eyes.

The nadis can be classified into the following two groups.

1. Pranavaha nadi which carry vital energy
2. Manovaha nahi which carry mental energy (manas shakti).

Just as electricity flow through complex circuits, prana also flows throughout the entire mind - body complex through the nadis. As per the yogic philosophy , 72,000 nadis are perceived to be in the astral body (refer section 43 of part three). Fourteen of these nadis considered to be very important are clubbed into the following three groups. They are perceived to originate from the base of the spine, follow the course of the sushumna and branch out at certain points along the spine and then terminate at the sensory organs (ear, nose, eyes, tongue and skin), hands, feet and perennial areas.

1. Nadis corresponding to the right side of the body: Pingala, pusha, payasvini and yashasvati.
2. Nadis corresponding to the left side of the body: Ida, shankhini, gandhari, and hastijihva.
3. Nadis corresponding to the central body: Alambusha, kuhu, vishvodhara, varuna, sarasvati, and sushumna

33. NADIS ON RIGHT & LEFT SIDE OF THE BODY

Following are some of the important nadis corresponding to the right side of the body.

Pingala nadi: It emanates from the right side of mooladhara chakra at the base of the spine, carries prana, spirals across the spinal cord in a criss cross way and terminates at the right nostril. Prana vayu flows through pingala.

Pusha nadi: Prana flowing through pusha nadi branches out from the third eye (between the eye brows) and terminates at right eye. Prana vayu flows through pusha nadi.

Payasvini nadi: Carrying prana it branches out from the third eye and terminates at the right ear.

Yashasvati Nadi: It branches out from navel and supplies prana to the right foot and right hand and terminates primarily in the thumb and the big toe.

Following are some of the important nadis corresponding to the left hand side of the body.

Ida nadi: It emanates from the left side of mooladhara chakra at the base of the spine, spirals across the sushumna in a criss cross way, carries the apana vayu and terminates at the left nostril.

Shankhini nadi: It branches out from the third eye, carries prana and terminates at the left ear.

Hastajivha nadi: It branches out from navel chakra, supplies prana to the left foot and the left hand and terminates at the tip of the left thumb and the tip of the left big toe.

Gandhari nadi: It branches out from the third eye, carries prana and terminates at the left eye.

34. NADIS IN THE CENRAL BODY

Following are some of the important nadis corresponding to the central body.

Sushumna nadi: It moves from the base of the spine to the crown of the head, up the centre of the spine. Kundalini shakti when awakened, moves through the sushumna, crosses all the chakras before uniting with the shiva shakti at the shahasrara. Flow of prana through sushumna signals a person's spiritual journey.

Alambusha nadi: It moves from the base of the spine, supplies energy to the organs of elimination and terminates at anus. Apana vayu moves through it.

Kuhu nadi: It flows from the base of the spine to the swadhisthana chakra and forward, supplies prana to the reproductive organs as well as to the urinary organs connected to them and terminates at the sex organs. Apana vayu runs through it.

Vishvodhara nadi: It moves from the base of the spine, supplies prana to the digestive system and terminates at the navel. Samana vayu runs through it.

Varuna nadi: It runs from the base of the spine to the heart chakra and supplies energy to the entire body, generally through the respiratory, circulatory and sebaceous systems and terminates at the skin. Vyana vayu flows through it.

Sarasvati nadi: It branches out from the throat chakra, moves, supplies energy to the mouth and throat area and terminates at the mouth. Udana vayu flows through it.

Nadis are connected to different locations in the body identified as chakras from where prana is distributed to different parts of the mind – body complex.

Out of the fourteen important nadis mentioned above, ida, pingala and sushumna plays the most significant part in human body.

35. IDA, PINGALA & SUSHUMNA NADI

Amongst all the nadis in the right hand side, left hand side and central part of the body as mentioned above, ida, pingala and sushumna nadi play the major and the most significant role in terms of physical, mental and spiritual well being of a person. All of these nadis move upwards from the same location in the perineum, the space between anal outlet and the genital outlet in the physical body. Starting from the base of the spinal cord,

1. the sushumna nadi moves straight up,
2. the ida nadi moves from the left side and spirals across the sushumna forming a criss cross pathway and terminates at the left side of the sushumna at a location in level with the place between the two eyebrows in the forehead.
3. the pingala nadi moves from the right side and spirals across the sushumna in the same way as that of the ida but in the opposite direction and terminates at the right side of the sushumna at a location on in level with the place between two eyebrows in the forehead.

The perceived flow patterns of ida, pingala and sushumna nadi is shown in figure no. 11.

FLOW PATTERS OF PINGALA, IDA & SUSHUMNA NADI

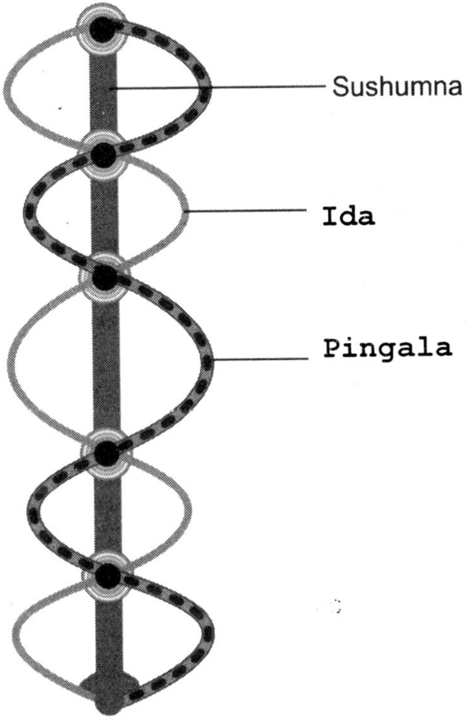

Figure no. 11

At the physical level, ida nadi flows through the left nostril and pingala nadi flows through the right nostril. At any point in time, the flow is always more in one nostril than the other. This phenomenon continues at regular and periodical intervals throughout the whole day. When the prominence of flow continues through ida and pingala nadi (alternately), a person remains busily engaged in worldly activities. When sushumna (which normally lies dormant) starts operating, the person becomes dead to the world and is said to be on way to his spiritual consciouness.

36. CHAKRAS

Like nadis, the chakras are also subtle in nature and are visible only to those who have developed psychic vision. They are the key central points at specific locations of the body from where the prana is distributed to different organs in different parts of the body. There are numbers of chakras out of which seven are considered to be major. These seven chakras are aligned with the sushumna, and are connected by three important nadis - ida, pingala and sushumna.

How the Ida, pingala and sushumna nadis move upwards from the same location in the perineum, the space between the anal outlet and the genital outlet in the physical body has been discussed in section 35 and shown in figure no. 12 figure no. 11. In their upwards movements, the three nadis of reference meet each other at six different points. These meeting points are the locations of the first six major chakras. Starting from the base and moving upwards along the sushumna, the successive chakras are identified as

1. mooladhara chakra,
2. swadhisthana chakra,
3. manipura chakra,
4. anahata chakra,
5. vishudhi chakra and
6. ajna chakra.

Beyond ajna chakra, the sushumna extends further upwards and terminates at the crown of the head. This location is known as shahasrara, the seventh chakra. Shahasrara is also known as an abode of highest consciousness. The flow patterns of ida, pingala and sushumna nadi and the locations of the different chakras in the subtle body are shown in figure no. 12.

Ida, Pingala & Sushumna nadi and
the seven major Chakras

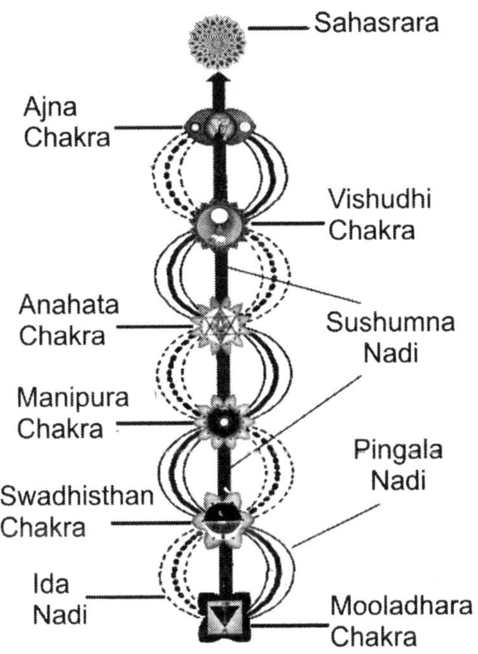

Fig. no. 12

37. CHARACTERISTICS OF THE CHAKRAS

Energy flows in and out of the body through the chakras. The function of the chakras is to spin and draw in prana and distribute it to different parts of the body to keep the spiritual, mental, emotional and physical health of the body in balance. The spinning action of the chakras put the prana into flow patterns through the nadis. Chakras function like transformers. Through the nadis they receive various forms of prana and transform them into the frequencies needed by different areas of physical bodies for their sustenance and development. Each chakra is a switch with unique attributes and characteristics and is capable of activating specific areas of the brain.

Chakras are represented by lotus flower which is a symbol of purity and resurrection. In spite of growing in unclear and muddy water, lotus flower always blossoms into a pure and untainted flower. Symbolization of chakras with lotus flower depicts that growth of a person even from the lowest state of awareness to the highest state of consciousness is possible.

Each chakra is represented by specific number of petals. Number of petals indicate the energy or the vibrational frequency of a specific chakra. More the number of petals in the chakra, higher is the frequency of energy that particular chakra is attuned to. An imbalance in the chakra results in physical and mental illness and finds expression through specific human physical systems.

Status of unfolding of the petals symbolizes a person's state of consciousness. Closed, partially opened and fully opened petals reflect a person's different stages of inner consciousness i.e. ignorance, aspiration and illumination that he must pass through in his quest for spiritual enlightenment. Ideally chakras should all be open and active (neither underactive nor overactive nor closed). Concentrating on the chakras, when specific breathing practices are applied, the chakras can be opened and activated.

38. CHAKRAS ROTATE

The chakras are constantly in a state of motion. That is why they are called chakras which in sanskrit means 'wheel'. It is the rotation which attracts energy and draws it in or gives it out, depending on the direction of rotation.

Generally, depending on the sex of a person, the chakras rotate either in clockwise or in anti-clockwise direction. For example, if the chakra in a man is rotating clockwise; the same chakra in a woman will rotate in counter clockwise and vice versa. This could be one of the reasons of the magnetic pull between man and woman that enable their energies to complement each other. Chakras are centers of overall consciousness, perceptions, emotions, thoughts and ideas. The moment a person starts doing things which are different with respect to the core nature of the specific chakra, the spin direction can change. Spinning speed is lowest at mooladhara and swadhisthana chakra. It increases from the manipura chakra onwards and is highest in the ajna chakra.

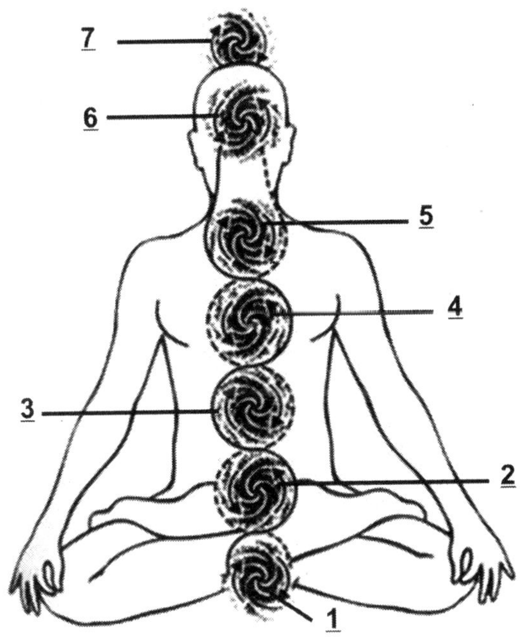

Figure no. 13

The direction in which a chakra rotates varies from chakra to chakra. Each chakra rotates in a different direction as shown in figure no. 13 (1 = Mooladhara, 2 = Swadhisthana, 3 = Manipura, 4 = Anahata, 5 = Vishudhi, 6 = Ajna, 7 = Shahasrara).

Every clockwise direction is primarily male in nature (which is in accordance with the Chinese teaching YANG). It represents will power and activities characterized by aggression and force. Every counter clockwise rotation is female in nature (this is in accordance with the Chinese teachings YING). Every counter clockwise direction represents receptiveness and agreement as well as the characteristics of weakness in every sphere of life.

39. SYNTHESIS OF CHAKRAS WITH ENDOCRINE GLANDS

There is a synthesis of the chakras with the endocrine glands. Each chakra corresponds to an endocrine gland. Physically the endocrine system is a collection of hormone-producing glands and cells located in various parts of the body. Hormones are complex chemical substances that are secreted in to the bloodstream. The endocrine glands secrete hormones directly into the blood stream, which carries them to other parts of the body where they regulate the continuous and prolonged functions of growth and development, cellular metabolism, puberty, reproduction, body water, tissues, body's defenses against stress etc.

When secretion of hormones is low, brain development stagnates, slow and deep breath, intake of prana in the body increases. This leads to rise in the level of secretion from the endocrine glands to the blood stream. Details of chakras and their corresponding associated organs and glands are mentioned below in table no. 5.

CHAKRAS	ASSOCIATED ORGANS	ENDOCRINE GLANDS
Shasrara	Upper brain, right eye	Pineal
Ajna	Ears, nose, lower brain, nervous system, left eye	Pituitary
Vishudhi	Lungs, larynx, alimentary canal (pathway by which food enters the body and solid wastes are expelled – mouth, intestines, anus etc.)	Thyroid, parathyroid
Anahata	Heart, blood, circulatory system	Thymus
Manipura	Stomach, gall bladder, liver	Pancreas
Swadhisthana	Reproductive system, spleen	Testes, ovaries
Mooladhara	Spinal column, kidneys	Adrenals

Table no. 5

All of the chakras and glands are of equal importance. When one chakra is out of balance it affects the energy flow creating blockage in the flow through other chakras. Concentrating on the activation of the chakras through specific breathing practices therefore is of great importance.

40. DESCRIPTION OF THE SEVEN MAJOR CHAKRAS

Mooladhara chakra: It is also popularly known as root chakra. It is located at the perineum (the space between the anal outlet and the genital outlet). When this chakra is inactive, it causes number of diseases and when it is over-active, people become materialistic, greedy, obsessed with being secure and resist change. Mooladhara chakra

1. controls human physical energies required for everyday survival,
2. is associated with adrenal glands,
3. is represented by four rose petals of red colour,
4. is related to the element earth.

Mooladhara chakra is the seat of the primal energy, the Kundalini Shakti. Physically, mooladhara governs sexuality, mentally it governs stability, emotionally it governs sensuality, and spiritually it governs a sense of security.

The manifestation and development of human consciousness begins from here, passes through the other chakras before moving upwards toward the shahasrara chakra. Apana vayu is the source of power for mooladhara chakra.

Swadhisthana chakra is located below the navel and just above the genital organ. This chakra is

1. responsible for the purification of body fluids flowing through kidneys, bladder and lymph,
2. associated with ovaries, testes and prostrate glands,
3. represented by six number of rose petals of orange colour,
4. related to the element water.

Physically, swadisthana chakra governs reproduction, mentally it governs creativity, emotionally it governs joy, and spiritually it governs enthusiasm. People with active swadhisthana energy are normally fluid, spontaneous but can be very unpredictable at times. This chakra has a very strong influence upon human moods and emotional energies like sex. Vyana vayu is the source of power for the swadhisthana chakra.

Manipura chakra is situated in the spine just below the navel. Physically, manipura governs digestion, mentally it governs personal power, emotionally it governs expansiveness, and spiritually it governs all matters of growth. If this chakra is under-active, people suffer from sluggishness or malfunctions of the digestive system. If this chakra is over-active, people become domineering and sometimes even aggressive. Manipura chakra

1. is chiefly associated with the process of digestion and metabolism
2. governs the functioning of the gastric glands, the pancreas, gall bladder etc. which produce and secrete enzymes, acids and juices necessary for digestion and absorption of the nutrients.
3. is represented by ten number of rose petals with yellow colour.
4. is associated with the element agni or fire.

Manipura chakra is also known as the chakra of will power and human connection to dream world. Samana vayu is the source of power for the manipura chakra.

Anahata chakra is situated in the spine behind the sternum, in level with the heart. It is –

1. a chakra of love and compassion and controls human mental energies (emotions, feelings etc.).
2. associated with thymus glands
3. represented by twelve number of lotus petals in green colour.
4. represented by element air.

Physically Anahata governs circulation, emotionally it governs unconditional love for the self and others, mentally it governs passion and spiritually it governs devotion. Since air represents freedom and expansion, it signifies that in this chakra human consciousness can expand into infinity. Prana vayu is the source energy of anahata chakra.

Vishudhi chakra is situated at the throat. Physically, vishuddha governs communication, emotionally it governs independence, mentally it governs fluency and spiritually it governs a sense of security. If this chakra is inactive, people will get cold, cough, thyroid problem and lack of communication skills. If this chakra is over-active, people tend to speak too much, usually to domineer and keep others at a distance.

Vishudhi chakra

1. controls human spiritual energies and governs the vocal cords, the regions of the larynx, the thyroids and the parathyroid glands,
2. is associated with thyroid and parathyroid glands,
3. is represented by sixteen lotus petals of blue colour
4. corresponds to the element aakash (ether).

Vishudhi is known as a chakra of creativity and expression. Blockage of this chakra produces feelings of anxiety, lack of freedom associated with unfounded manifestations of swallowing problems and speech impediments. Udana vayu is the source of power in the vishudhi chakra.

Ajna chakra also known as the 'third eye' is located in between the eyebrows in the forehead. This is the centre where wisdom and intuition develop. If this chakra is inactive, a person will have negative thoughts, lack of energy which would make more bad karmas. If this chakra is over-active, the person may live in a world of fantasy way too much; in extreme cases hallucinations are possible. He who concentrates at this centre destroys all the karmas of the past lives. The benefits that are derived by meditation on this chakra cannot be described in words. Ajna chakra is

1. a chakra of perception and higher knowledge and represents the visual, intuitive and psychic center of perception,
2. associated most often with pituitary gland,
3. represented by ninety six numbers of lotus petals of purple colour.

Stimulation of ajna chakra leads to development of all the faculties of mind, like intelligence, memory, concentration etc. When ajna chakra is active, it is possible to send and receive thought transmission through this center.

Shahasrara chakra is located at the crown of the head. On physical level, shahasrara chakra is related to the pineal gland. The pineal gland is a light sensitive gland that produces the hormone melatonin which regulates sleep and awakening. Its proper functioning helps to improve thinking power and intelligence. It is large in children, but shrinks at puberty. It symbolizes detachment from illusion; an essential element in obtaining supramental consciousness of the truth that 'one is all and all is one'.

Sahasrara chakra is the last milestone of the evolution of human awareness. Shahasrara chakra is –

1. the abode of the highest spiritual consciousness, within which there is neither object nor subject,
2. associated most often with pineal gland,
3. represented by one thousand numbers of white lotus petals.

PART THREE

BREATH, PRANA & SPIRITUALITY

The subtle flow of prana through three important nadis – ida, pingala and sushumna play vital roles in human life especially in the spiritual field. The ida and pingala nadis are directly connected to the left and right nostrils respectively. Flow of prana through them influences human personality as well as nervous systems. Generally for most of the people, prana flows through ida and pingala nadi with sushumna nadi practically remaining dormant. At any point of time, the flow of prana is more either through ida or through pingala nadi. This trend alternates at regular intervals throughout the day.

Under normal circumstances, the flow of prana through ida and pingala nadis are involuntary, they however can be made to function voluntarily. Adapting specific asana and technique of breathing, when the flow of prana through ida and pingala are made equal and balanced, flow through sushumna commences. When the flow of prana through sushumna commences, it signals a person's start of journey in the spiritual path.

To move ahead in spiritual journey, activation of the sushumna and chakras are mandatory before the kundalini shakti is awakened. Once awakened, the kundalini shakti moves through sushumna, passes through the active chakras and meets the shiva shakti at the shahasrara. When this happens, a person attains spiritual enlightenment. In order to achieve this state, resorting only to specific asana and breathing techniques however is not enough. The person must also direct his whole life towards everything good; he must be free from hatred, greed, anger, envy, jealousy, passion and dependency. He must live in love, harmony and understanding with the environment.

41. SUBTLE BODIES

Beyond the tangible human physical body, there are five layers of bodies, each precisely fitting into the other. The totality of human body completes with these five different and distinct layers of bodies which have exclusive attributes and functions. The outermost layer is the material body within which the pranic body fits in. Pranic body, through which the prana flows in the form of vayus is the source of physical life. Inside the pranic body fits the mental body which governs all the mental activities and emotions. Deep within the mental body fits the intellectual body which has the power of discrimination that helps in decisions making. Inside the intellectual body lies the inner most layers called the bliss body. Bliss body is associated with the state of thoughtlessness where nothing matters, neither joy nor sorrow. This layer veils the atman, the supreme self.

The bodies mentioned above envelope the atman as different layers one over the other; that is why they are known as sheaths or koshas. The material body is known as annamaya kosha, the pranic body as pranamaya kosha, the mental body as manamaya kosha, the intellectual body as vijnanamaya kosha and bliss body as anandamaya kosha.

Only the outermost and the densest of the koshas i.e. the material body or the annamaya kosha is made of matter. Others are in the form of energy and are invisible to the physical eye. They are all **subtle bodies**; their presence however can be perceived and felt inside when close attention is given. All these subtle bodies can be strengthened and toned up through specific asana and breathing practices.

42. DESCRIPTION OF THE SHEATHS/KOSHAS

Annamaya kosha (material body): This is the outermost and the densest sheath of the human existence. It emerges from food assimilated in the form of semen by the father and is nourished in the womb by food taken by the mother. It continues to exist because of food consumed and ultimately after death of a person goes back to fertilizing the earth and becomes food again. In view of the above this sheath is called **annamaya kosha** (anna meaning food). It is also known as the **physical body** . Annamaya kosha consisting of flesh, bone, fat, muscles, physical organs, respiratory, circulatory and nervous system etc. grows in youth and decays in old age. It develops when good nourishing food is given, and decays if food is withdrawn, or if there is some disease.

Pranamaya kosha (pranic body): Prana, the vital energy flows through the pranic body via the nadis and chakras and circulates throughout the body. This sheath of energy because of being directly connected to prana, is called **pranamaya kosha**. It is responsible for holding the material body together. It governs all the biological processes from breathing to digestion and also controls bodily and spiritual rhythms. When prana stops functioning, hcart, lungs stop working and all the cells in the body begin to disintegrate. Specific breathing practices like pranayamas in yoga aim at replenishing as well as enhancing the vitality of the pranayama kosha.

Manamaya kosha (mental body): This sheath deals with the emotional, mental and perceptual part of the body, which comprises not just the mind, but also the organs within the body. It processes input from the five senses and responds reflexively through gnyanendriyas and karmendriyas on day to day basis. It is the sheath where a person moves from physical feeling and rhythm to emotional feeling. Since this sheath deals with the mental aspects, it is also known as **manamaya kosha**. While pranamaya kosha functions continuously, the manamaya kosha can function intermittently. For example, when a person is sleeping, his senses (manaamaya kosha) are nonfunctional, but he still continues to breathe (pranamaya kosha functioning).

Vijnanamaya kosha (intellectual body): This sheath represents the intelligence or consciousness which is the discriminating part of the mind. Since it is associated with judgment and discernment, it is known as **vijnanamaya kosha**. Manamaya kosha is the gross level of mind that comprises of emotions, thoughts and different types of feelings; it however does not have the capacity to discriminate between right and wrong or good and bad. Vijnanamaya on the other hand embraces all the functions of the higher mind like awareness, insight, consciousness etc. Emotions left unchecked by awareness can be destructive. This sheath governs the gross mind (manamaya kosha) to take appropriate decisions with knowledge accrued from various sources through different means.

Anandamaya kosha (bliss body): This sheath is the subtlest of the bodies and is said to be the source of ananda and is known as anandamaya kosha. Truly speaking anandamaya kosha signifies a state when there is no happiness and no unhappiness. In happiness, a person jumps; in unhappiness he becomes morose. In both the circumstances, the mind swings. In ananda, there is no swinging of mind. In this sheath, a person drops from conscious awareness into the state of pure and radiant bliss (spiritual bliss); in this state he fails to express himself but enjoys an unified experience and that experience does not change with circumstances or environment. A bliss body generally remains under developed for vast majority of people. Bliss body is also known as casual body.

Specific asana and breathing practice helps a person to create a track and access the deeper koshas. Asana prepares the outer body; specific breathing practices activate the activities of the pranic body and help in controlling the fluctuating emotional state of the mind. The five koshas surrounding the atman, the supreme self is shown in figure no. 14.

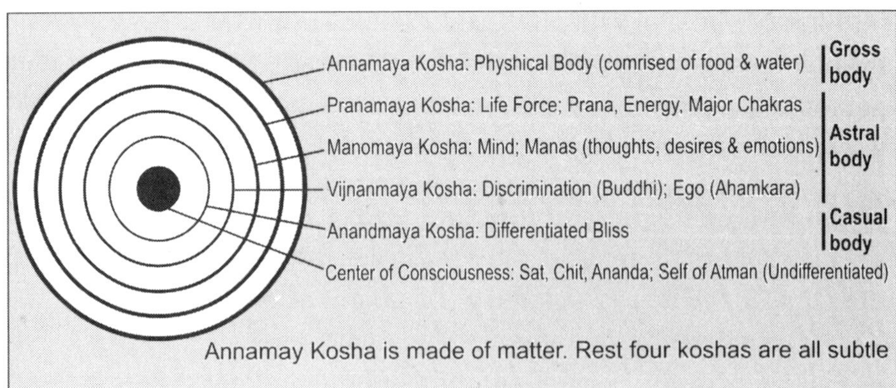

Figure no.14

43. GROSS, ASTRAL & CASUAL BODY

The five koshas are divided into the following classifications.

1. Gross body (sthula sharira)
2. Astral boy (linga sharira)
3. Casual body (karana sharira)

It is the energy that threads the physical, astral and casual body. When the energy starts to penetrate into each layer, a person begins to feel the sense of integration of his entire being.

Gross body is the physical body that is made up of five elements earth, air, fire, water and ether (refer section 57 of part three), and is subjected to six fold changes – birth, subsistence, growth, maturity, decay and death. Annamaya kosha and part of pranamaya kosha (physical manifestation) reside in the gross body. At death the physical body perishes and its five constituent elements are dissolved back into the respective elements in nature.

Astral body is where the mind and the intellect live. Manomaya kosha and vijnanamaya kosha and part of pranamaya kosha reside in astral body. They are communicated through a network of energy centers (chakras) within the astral spine or sushumna nadi and connected by pranic pathways or nadis. The astral body is a person's personal dream vehicle. Dreams are the play ground of thought forms and thought forms are the precursors of future reality.

Causal body is not formed by anything physical; it requires energy to be transformed from the astral body to reach this layer. Anandmaya Kosh resides in causal body. Casual body is the doorway to the higher consciousness. It links individual consciousness with the collective consciousness. Causal body is the time keeper of the experience of a person's past soul. When a person dies, the essence of his life experience gets recorded in his casual body. Every time a person reincarnates, the causal history gets imprinted into his new physical and subtle bodies to affect his new life. That is how soul patterns are passed between lifetimes.

The gross, astral and casual bodies have no existence without atman, the self.

44. ATMAN THE SOUL

Sat, chit and ananda mentioned in figure no. 14 is translated as sat meaning truth, existence or pure being, chit meaning consciousness and ananda meaning bliss. That which exists in the past, present and future, which has no beginning, middle and end, is unchanging, is not conditioned in time, space and causation, exists during jagrat, swapna and sushupti, that which is the nature of one homogeneous essence is sat. Sat, chit and ananda are not three distinct entities. They are coeval and coexistent with atman. Just as water, jal, pani signify one and the same thing, same way sat-chit-ananda signify the one atman too. Sat is chit. Sat is ananda. Chit is sat. Chit is ananda. Ananda is sat. Ananda is chit. A person cannot split up sat-chit-ananda into three separate entities, just as he cannot separate light, heat and luminosity from fire.

Atman is the soul, the individualized unit of consciousness emanating from the Brahman. He who has realized sat, chit and ananda i.e. his atman is an emancipated person, he has nothing more to learn, has nothing more to do, has nothing more to gain. All his desires are gratified. He has obtained all worlds, he is freed from the jaws of death and has attained immortality.

Talking about atman, Swami Sivananda said, "It has no physical or mental dimension as such, other than as a mere reflection or an idea in the mind. But unquestionably He exists and he alone is real. All else is false and withers away, crushed by the weight of sins and pressures of time". He further said, "The atman or the self is the silent partner of all human deeds and experiences, the observer and the indweller of all embodied beings. Its nature cannot be explained or described in human language adequately, as it is beyond the sense of the mind. It can only be experienced when all the-

1. sensory activities ceases to impact the mind,
2. when the mind itself is freed from the movements of thoughts and sense objects,
3. torment of desires, which are the prime cause of all human activity and suffering, subside to quietude."

A person experiences his self when his mind and the five senses are stilled and when the intellect is also stilled. Through specific breathing practices, a person can attain complete stillness in which he can enter that state of oneness. It is meditation under the guidance of a guru that leads a person to realize his self, the atman.

In the subsequent sections, breathing and regulation of the flow of prana through ida, pingala and sushumna nadi and the activation of the dormant kundalini shakti to achieve spiritual enlightenment has been discussed.

45. CONNECTION OF NOSTRILS TO IDA & PINGALA NADIS

Ida and pingala nadi play significant roles in the movement of pranic energy in the human system. The flow of energy through ida and pingala have their own characteristics. While prana vayu circulates inside pingala, the apana circulates inside Ida. The Ida and Pingala nadis are often referred to the two hemispheres of the brain. Each Hemisphere has different qualities and stimulates mankind in diverse ways (refer section 46 of part three).

At physical level, ida is connected to the left nostril and pingala is connected to the right nostril. The flow of prana through individual nostril at any point of time can be gauged by measuring the flow of breath in the nostrils. Under normal circumstances, or at any point of time, the flow always measures more in one nostril than the other. This pattern of one nostril flow domination alternates between the two nostrils at regular intervals throughout the day. Though the flow of energy through ida and pingala are involuntary, if a person so desires, he can consciously influence them by adapting specific breathing practices.

46. CHARACTERISTICS OF 'FLOW' THRO' IDA & PINGALA NADI

Dominance of the flow of prana through ida and pingala nadi have marked influence on human personality. When the 'flow' through the left nostril is more i.e. when the flow of prana through ida nadi is dominating, a person is able to concentrate hard, think and manage his emotions better and take up any kind of mental work. Ida nadi regarded as the lunar or chandra (moon) nadi is cool and nurturing by nature and is said to control all mental processes and the feminine aspects of human personality. Ida nadi corresponds to the left hand side of the body and the right hand side of the brain. With right hand side of the brain dominating, a person is generally said to be more intuitive, thoughtful and subjective. However, if this dominance of flow on the left nostril continues for a longer time, beyond the normal schedule specific to a person, it creates imbalances in his mental work.

When the 'flow' through the right nostril is more i.e. when flow of prana through pingala nadi is dominating, a person is able to do more physical work, digest food and take up any kind of physical work. Flow of energy through pingala encourages growth of the body. Pingala nadi regarded as the solar or surya (sun) nadi is warm and stimulating by nature and is said to control all vital somatic processes (i.e. processes that has to do with the body rather than the mind) and oversee the masculine aspects of human personality. Pingala nadi corresponds to the right hand side of the body and the left hand side of the brain. With left hand side of the brain dominating, a person generally is said to be more logical, analytical, and objective. However, if the right nostril continues to flow for a longer period, beyond the normal schedule specific to a person, it creates imbalances in the flow of pranic current in the body.

It is to be noted that the masculine and feminine aspects of human personality mentioned above have no relation to sex. When flow through ida nadi is prominent, even a man can have some of the feminine aspects predominant in him. Likewise, when flow through pingala nadi is prominent, even a woman can have some of the masculine aspects predominant in her. Relevant features of ida nadi and pingala nadi are summarized in table no. 6.

PARTICULARS	IDA	PINGALA
Prominence of flow of breath	Left nostril	Right nostril
Effect on body temperature	Cooling	Hot
Nature of human personality	Female	Male
Abilities to do mental/ physical activities	More of mental	More of physical
Characteristic resembling planet	Moon	Sun
Corresponding autonomic nervous system	Parasympathetic	Sympathetic

Table no. 6

An ida dominated person may be very nurtured and calm , but he is more susceptible to depression, exhaustion and extreme introversion. On the other hand, a pingala dominated person may be full of creativity and vitality, yet he is more anxious and restless.

Flow of prana through ida and pingala nadi have direct relation to human nervous system.

47. IDA & PINGALA NADI RELATES TO NERVOUS SYSTEM

Flow of energy through ida and pingala nadis have marked influence on the human nervous system which embraces the brain and the spinal cord along with emanating nerves. The human nervous system can broadly be divided into two main systems – central nervous system (CNS) and peripheral nervous system (PNS). Central nervous system embraces the brain and the spinal cord, and the peripheral nervous system embraces the entire nervous system outside the brain and the spinal cord. Some of these nerves gather information while others transmit orders. Peripheral nervous system functions through two sub systems - somatic nervous system and autonomic nervous system.

Somatic nervous system is responsible for movement of voluntary muscles. This system carries nerve impulses back and forth between the central nervous system, which is the brain and the spinal cord, and the skeletal muscles, skin, and sensory organs. It embraces the following nerves

1. sensory nerves – these nerves carry messages to the brain and spinal cord from the body,
2. motor nerves – these nerves carry messages from brain and spinal cord to the body,
3. connecting or mixed nerves – these nerves carry both sensory as well as motor nerves.

Autonomic nervous system functions involuntarily and reflexively. It helps the body to react in times of emergency. It is again divided into two systems - sympathetic nervous system and parasympathetic nervous system.

The sympathetic nerves stimulate and accelerate the automatic function of the nerves and help a person to prepare and face life threatening emergencies and challenges, and are responsible for

1. increase in heart beat rate,
2. increase in respiration rate,
3. increase in blood pressure
4. decrease in digestive system activities,
5. intensification of the efficiency of the eyes, ears and other sense organs.

Obviously, nobody wants to be in the above stressful state for long.

Nerves of the parasympathetic nervous system retards or inhibits all automatic functions of the nerves. They directly oppose the sympathetic nerves and are responsible for

1. decrease in heart beat rate,
2. decrease in respiration rate,
3. decrease in blood pressure
4. increase in digestive system activities,
5. conservation of energy.

The schematic details of the human nervous systems are shown in table no. 7.

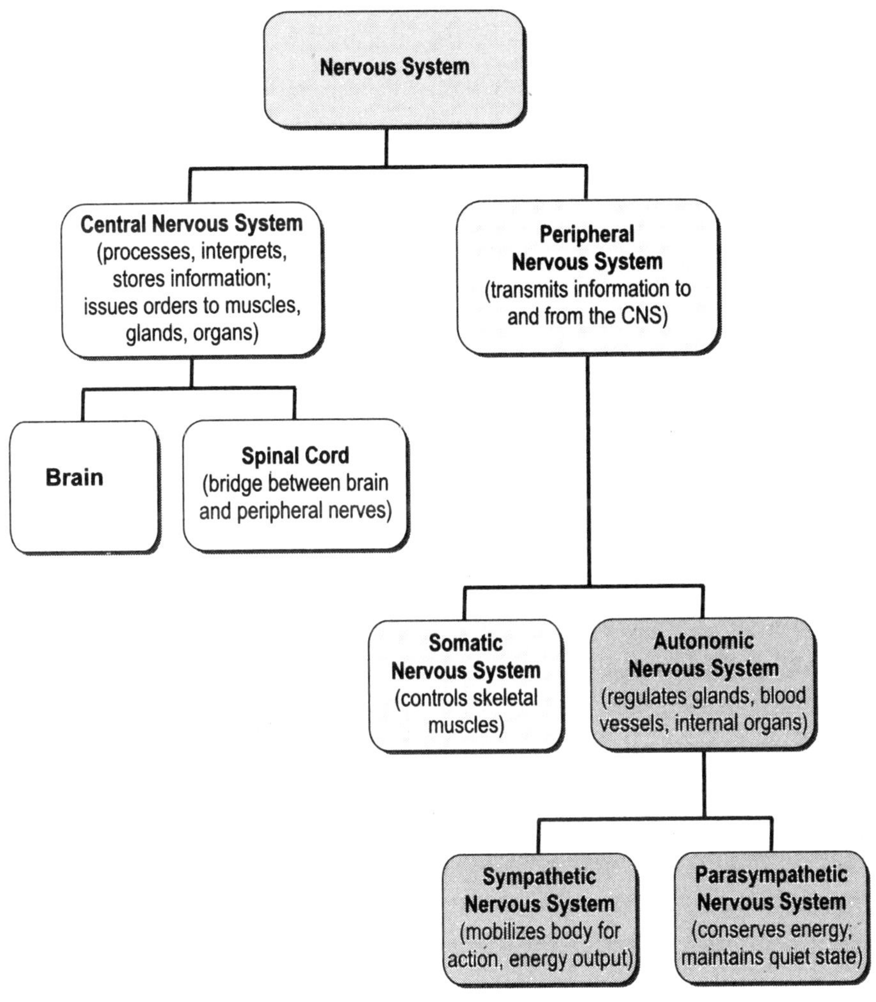

Table no. 7

At the physical level, ida and pingala correspond to the two aspects of the autonomic nervous system - the sympathetic and parasympathetic.

Pingala coincides with the sympathetic nervous system and ida with the parasympathetic nervous system.

48. FLOW THROUGH IDA & PINGALA NADI CAN BE REVERSED

Though the dominance of flow of prana through ida and pingala alternate at regular intervals throughout the day, it is generally observed that when there is surge of emotions, the pingala nadi becomes more dominant, and with emotions subsiding, the ida nadi becomes more dominant. During rapid and frequent vacillations in the emotional state, prominence of the flow of two nadis also vacillates. However, in such a situation, pingala nadi always plays the dominant role more. In an emotional person, this roller coaster of emotions continues in the subconscious mind even during sleeping hours. This is because the impressions in the sub-conscious mind is active even during sleep.

If the natural cycle of alternate dominant flow patterns of ida and pingala nadi get disturbed for any reason, body chemistry changes and a person's physical, emotional and mental state starts getting affected. For example, when a person sleeps at night, generally his ida nadi is dominant; however, if instead his pingala nadi becomes dominant during this period, he experiences restlessness and finds it difficult to sleep. Likewise, if the ida is prominent when a person is eating food, his digestive system gets affected causing indigestion.

Flow of prana through ida and pingala is completely involuntary; however, by adapting appropriate breathing practices, it is possible to consciously influence them at will and if necessary alter their flow patterns. When flow through ida is predominant and there is physical work to be done, it is possible to redirect the flow of the breath to pingala and obtain the necessary energy. Likewise, if at any point of time, mental work is to be done, the energy can be redirected to flow through ida from pingala. By regulating and balancing the flow of prana through ida and pingala, a person can create

1. a balanced wholeness in his overall personality
2. an opening for the prana to flow through sushumna.

49. DESCRIPTION OF SUSHUMNA NADI

It has been mentioned earlier that sushumna nadi starts from the bottom of the spine at mooladhara chakra and extends up to the shahasrara chakra at the crown of the head. Sushumna, the hollow passageway of prana as vayu is the astral spine i.e. the spine of the energy body (refer pranamaya kosha in section 42 of part three).

There is a hollow canal inside the physical spinal cord known as canalis centralis. Originating from the mooladhara chakra, the sushumna nadi runs upward inside the canalis centralis, pierces the upper palate i.e. the roof of the mouth and finally bifurcates into two branches - anterior and posterior. While the anterior branch is routed towards the place between the eye brows (ajna chakra) and from there moves to brahmarandhra, the posterior branch passes from behind the head and joins the Brahmarandhra.

Sushumna encircles another nadi known as vajra nadi. Within vajra nadi, there is another nadi called chitra nadi. Vajra nadi and chitra nadi correspond to the two bodies called manomaya kosha and vijnanmaya kosha (refer section 41 of part three). Chitra nadi encircles another nadi known as brahma nadi. Brahma nadi is the subtlest of all nadis and is known as the spine of the casual body or anandamaya kosha (refer section 42 of chapter three). The lowest part of sushumna i.e the base of the brahma nadi is called the brahmadwara; it is the doorway of the awakened kundalini shakti in its journey towards the abode of the supreme self, at the crown of the head.

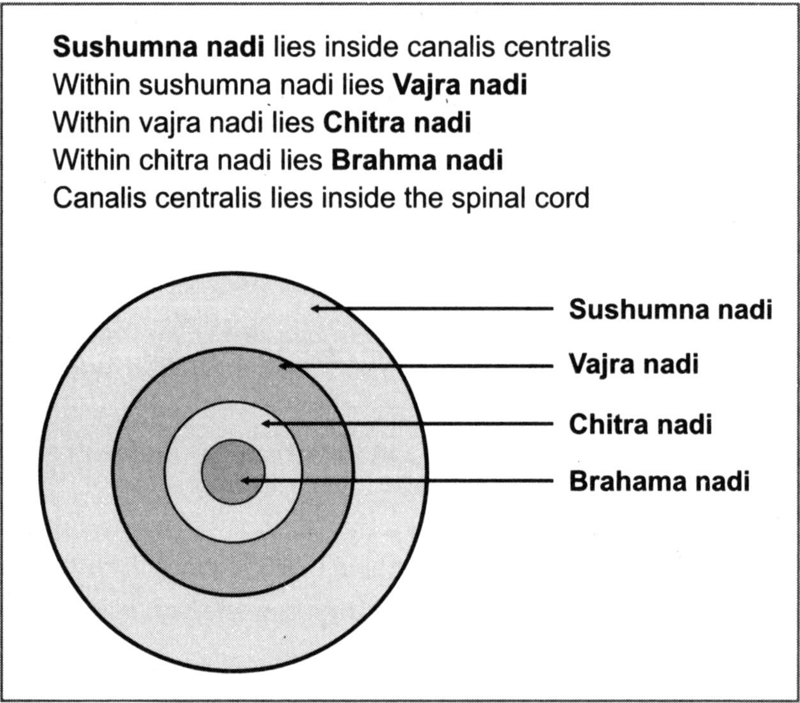

Figure no. 15

Since sushumna nadi contains the brahma nadi within, it is also known as brahma nadi. A schematic diagram of sushumna nadi is shown in figure no. 15.

50. WHAT HAPPENS WHEN SUSHUMNA NADI OPENS

It has been mentioned in section 48 of part three that through specific breathing practice a person can regulate, equalize and balance the flow of prana through ida and pingala nadi, and when this happens, flow of prana through sushumna commences. While flow of prana through ida stimulates the mental faculties and flow of prana through pingala stimulates the physical body, flow of prana through sushumna stimulates a person's spiritual potential.

It is a fact that during the periodic shifting of the prominence of 'flow' from ida nadi to pingala nadi and vice versa, flow of prana does get entry into the sushumna; but such periods are too small.

A person is busy and engaged in worldly activities as long as his breath continues to flow through Ida and Pingala. However, under the condition of equal and balanced flow of prana through ida and pingala nadi, when the prana flow gets directed towards sushumna nadi, all the mental distractions of the person gets removed; he becomes dead to the external world, and enters into a world which is full of peace and tranquility. The joy he derives during this period is unique; it cannot be compared to any sensory pleasure. A person entering this state never complains of dispersions of mind; his level of concentration improves. When this happens, the mind becomes steady. This steadiness of the mind is termed as "Unmani awastha". This state enables a person to sit in meditation for a longer period of time.

Most of the people in general are unaware of the importance of sushumna operation and its implications on physical, mental and spiritual life. As a result they breathe only through ida and pingala nadi leaving the sushumna nadi hardly utilized.

Equalizing and balancing the flow of prana through ida and pingala to create the condition for opening of the sushumna nadi warrants that the nadis are purified first. When the nadis are impure, breath cannot penetrate into the sushumna. There are various types of breathing practices through which nadis can consciously be purified, and the flow of prana through ida and pingala be equalized and balanced to create the opening for the sushumna nadi to flow. Such breathing practices in yoga are known as pranayamas. Pranayamas has cooling effect on the mind and body and aid in meditation.

51. PRANAYAMAS & MEDITATION

Concept of pranayama conveys wider meaning contrary to the general perception that it is a measure only to control breath. Pranayama is derived from the combination of two Sanskrit words – prana (the vital energy) and ayama (meaning extension or expansion). Pranayama embraces extension/ expansion of prana in the human body; it basically utilizes breathing to influence the flow of prana through the subtle nadis to different parts of the human body. Pranayama works mainly in the pranamaya kosha i.e. the energy body (refer section 41 of part three). It makes proper distribution of the five major prana vayus – prana vayu, apana vayu, samana vayu, udana vayu and vyana vayu (refer section 30 of part two) in the body.

As per ancient Indian philosopher Patanjali, pranayama is defined as the regulation of the incoming and outgoing flow of breath with the additional dimension of retention. Unlike normal breathing cycle, a cycle of pranayama therefore consists of three components–inhalation (puraka), exhalation (rechaka) and retention (kumbhaka).

Puraka and rechaka represent inhalation and exhalation respectively of a normal breath. While puraka involves application of energy with associated tensed muscles, during rechaka the tensed muscles get released. The additional act of retention i.e. holding of breath involved in pranayama is called kumbhaka. The 'retention' can be after puraka, after rechaka or after each puraka as well as each rechaka. The duration and the type of kumbhaka are dependent on the specific type of pranayama a person performs. Proper practice of inhalation and exhalation to strengthen the lungs and balance the nervous and pranic system is a prerequisite for a person before he can successfully learn the act of kumbhaka. The success of pranayama depends on the maintenance of proper balance between puraka, rechaka and kumbhaka. Pranayamas are proven breathing processes which enable a person to cool down his mind under different circumstances and guide him to attain the state of deep meditation. There are number of variations in the practice of pranayamas. Benefits arising from the practices of some of the common pranayamas are listed below. It is always desired that these breathing practices are learned under the guidance of an expert practitioner.

BHRAMARI PRANAYAMA: When a person undergoes stress arising out of cross thoughts, his buzzing mind can be calmed down and a break can be applied to his disturbing thought processes through the application of the breathing process known as bhramari pranayama. It enables a person to get relieved of his stress and cerebral tension, alleviate anger, anxiety and insomnia, and induce a meditative state by harmonizing the mind and directing his awareness inward. The humming sound produced during the practice has soothing effect on the mind and the nervous system. To perform bhramari pranayama, the following steps are involved:-

1. Sitting comfortably in a quiet and well ventilated place with eyes closed and hand resting on the knees with body fully relaxed.
2. The lips are to be kept gently closed with teeth slightly separated so that the sound vibrations are heard and felt distinctly throughout the period of practice.
3. With arms raised sideways and elbows bent, the hands are to be brought to the ears.
4. The index fingers or the middle fingers are to be used either to plug the ears by inserting the fingers in the ear hole or to press the ear flaps without inserting the fingers in the ear hole.
5. During inhalation and exhalation, the concentration always has to be on the ajna chakra (the place between the eye brows). Inhalation should be done through the nose.
6. After a deep inhalation, exhalation is to be done slowly in a controlled manner making all the way a deep, steady humming sound like that of a black bee. The humming has to be even and continuous during the entire period of exhalation. The sound needs to be soft and mellow to make the front of the skull reverberate.
7. At the end of the exhalation, the hands are to be returned to the knees and then raised again for the next breath. The above completes one round of breathing.

Five to ten rounds of breathing is good enough to start with. With time and practice this can be increased further. In case of extreme mental tension or anxiety, the practice can be increased to even thirty minutes.

To relieve mental tension, bhramari pranayama can be practiced at any time of the day; best time of practice however is early morning or late at night when the environment is noiseless.

KAPALBHATI PRANAYAMA: When a person feels low on energy, the breathing practice of kapalbhatti pranayama helps his energy to soar. This practice enables a person to energize and calm down his mind in preparation for meditation. Its energizing effect on his mind is such that he does not fall asleep while sitting on meditation. The practice also has cleansing effect on the lungs. Additionally, the process purifies the pranic nadis, removes sensory distractions, balances and strengthens the nervous system and tones the digestive systems. The practice of kapalbhati pranayama also known as frontal brain cleansing breath should be performed on an empty stomach or at least three to four hours after meals. Performing kapalbhati pranayama involves the following steps.

1. Sitting in a comfortable position, with head and spine in straight position with hands resting on the knees.
2. The focus always has to be on the flow of breath with eyes closed and body relaxed (without application of external force).
3. Exhalation has to be through both nostrils with a forceful contraction of the abdominal muscles. The following inhalation has to be taken passively by allowing the abdominal muscles to relax.
4. The inhalation has to be a spontaneous recoil, without involvement of any additional effort.
5. After completion of ten rapid breaths in succession, the inhalation and exhalation has to be made deeper. The breath then has to be allowed to return to normalcy.
6. The above completes one round of breathing. To start with at least five rounds of breaths must be practiced.
7. The rapid breathing has to be from the abdomen, with shoulder and face remaining in relaxed position. The beginners however can take free normal breaths between the rounds and increase their breath from ten counts to fifty counts once the abdominal muscles become stronger.

Kapalbhati pranayama should not be practiced by those suffering from heart disease, high blood pressure, vertigo, hernia or gastric ulcer. For women, it is not recommended during pregnancy.

UJJAYI PRANAYAMA: It helps in the soothing of the nervous system and calming of the mind. It is particularly beneficial for calming the mind of stress, insomnia, and mental tension. That is why it is also known as tranquillizing pranayama. It has a balancing influence on the entire cardio respiratory system and eases feelings of irritation and frustration. It has a profound relaxing effect at the psychic level.

To create the ujjayi breathing, a person must constrict the back of the throat while inhaling and exhaling through the nostrils with lips remaining gently closed. The process is associated with audible sound often compared to the sound of the ocean. That is why ujjayi breathing is also called "ocean breath". The name ujjayi is derived from the Sanskrit word "ujjayi," which means "to conquer" or "to be victorious". Ujjayi breathing therefore is also referred to as "victorious breath" or "hissing breath". During Ujjayi breathing the lower belly expands activating the Mooladhara and Sadhisthana chakras. After that the breath rises to the lower rib cage where it activates the Manipura and Anahata chakra. The air then moves to the upper chest and the throat before it comes out of the body through the nose. Ujjayi stretches the breath, warms the inhaled air before it enters the lungs and this warmth unlocks its powerful healing process. To perfom ujjayi pranayama the following steps are involved:-

1. Sitting in a comfortable position with eyes closed.
2. Concentrating on the nostrils; the breath should be allowed to become calm and rhythmic.
3. Concentration then has to be shifted to the throat with the imagination that breath is being drawn through throat not through nostrils.
4. As the breathing becomes slower and deeper, the glottis has to be gently contracted so that a soft snoring sound like 'HHHHAAAA' is produced in the throat.

5. It will be noticed that there is a spontaneous contraction of the abdomen, without any efforts being made.
6. Both inhalation and exhalation has to be long, deep and controlled and the sound from the throat should be audible to the practitioner.
7. The practice can start with ten breaths and then increased to five minutes. It can subsequently be enhanced to ten or twenty minutes.

Ujjayi breathing can be performed in any position, standing, sitting or lying. Those suffering from slip disc or vertebral spondylitis may seek expert practitioner's advice and perform it in vajrasana or makarasana.

BHASTRIKA PRANAYAMA: It is also called bellow breath as air is drawn forcefully in and out of the lungs like the bellows of a village blacksmith. It is helpful in increasing vitality and lowering the stress and anxiety levels, clearing the passages of pranaic flow and opening of sushumna nadi for prana to flow through it. It balances and strengthens the nervous system, induces peace, tranquility and one-pointedness of mind in preparation for meditation.

To perform bhastrika pranayama the following steps are involved:-

1. Sitting in a comfortable posture with hands placed on the knees.
2. Staying relaxed with focus on the breathing pattern with head and spine straight and whole body relaxed.
3. Taking a deep breath in and breathing out forcefully through the nose. Inhalation has to be forceful through both the nostrils making sure that the lungs are full with air. The exhalation also has to be done with application of force making a hissing sound. Forceful inhalation results from full expansion of the abdominal muscles and forceful exhalation from contraction of the abdominal muscles without straining.
4. How much force is to be applied during inhalation and exhalation is to be determined by the individual's health and endurance

power. Applied force is to be increased gradually by maintaining equal force of inhalation and exhalation.

5. During the entire period of practice, the abdomen is not to be blown up; instead the chest area should be blown up. During inhalation, the diapgragm descends and the abdomen moves outward. During exhalation, the diaphragm moves upward and the abdomen moves inward.
6. The practice is to be repeated for ten breaths to complete one round. Initially five rounds can be done.
7. The practice is to be performed every day. With acclimatization, breathing speed as well as numbers of rounds for practice can be gradually enhanced without compromising on rhythm.

Bhastrika pranayama should always be performed under the guidance of a proven practioner. Those who have high blood pressure or heart disease should not practice bhastrika pranayama.

NADI SHODHANA PRANAYAMA: It enables a person to reverse the periodic dominance of the flow of breath from ida nadi to pingala nadi and vice versa, at will and at any point of time. It ensures:-

1. nourishment of the whole body with extra supply of oxygen,
2. efficient expulsion of carbon dioxide,
3. removal of toxins from the body,
4. increase in vitality with lowering of stress and anxiety levels by harmonizing the flow of pranas,
5. clearance of blockages of pranic flow
6. balanced flow of prana through ida and pingala nadis, thereby causing sushumna nadi to get opened and start operating.

How to perform nadi shodhana pranaya is detailed in section 52 of part three.

MEDITATION: Unlike other creatures, human mind has the capacity to think, contemplate, create, analyze and grow. It however has the vulnerability of extremity of thoughts. The mind keeps wandering here and there with cross thoughts mostly embracing either the past or the future with very little tendency to remain focused in the present moment. The various types of pranayamas which aim at bringing the wavering mind to a state of calmness and dwell in the present moment is known as meditation.

Common people generally meditate with the expectation of reaping the benefits of mental and physical well being including reduction in stress, anxiety, lowering of blood pressure, boosting of immune systems etc. In the bigger canvas, a person through meditation however aims at achieving a state of thoughtlessness. It is rightly said, "Meditation has the potential to take the mind in a state of no agitation, no hesitation, no anticipation and no expectation". When such a state is achieved, a person's five senses gets stilled, his intellect gets stilled and he enters a state of oneness where there is no happiness and no unhappiness. In happiness, a person jumps; in unhappiness he becomes morose. In both the circumstances, the mind swings. In this state, there is no swinging of mind; a person simply gets transformed from conscious awareness into the state of pure and spiritual bliss. In this state a person fails to express himself but enjoys a unified experience and that experience does not change with circumstances or environment. Meditation is the path that leads towards spiritual consciousness.

52. ACTIVATION OF SUSHUMNA NADI

The application of nadi shodhana pranayama is a very common practice in the purification of nadis and opening of the sushumna nadi. Performing nadi shodhana pranayama warrants:-

1. sitting comfortably with spine in erect position and shoulders relaxed,
2. the left hand is to be placed on the left knee with the tip of the thumb gently touching the tip of index finger,
3. the tips of the index and middle fingers of the right hand are to be placed in between the eyebrows,
4. the ring and little finger of the right hand are to be placed on the left nostril (these two fingers will be used to open or close the left nostril),

5. the thumb of the right hand to be placed on the right nostril (this will be used for opening and closing of the right nostril).
6. Sitting in the above posture, the first step of a cycle of nadi shodhana pranayama involves closing of the right nostril with the thumb and breathing out through the left nostril. This is to be followed by breathing in through the left nostril with right nostril still closed by the thumb. Once it is done, the next step will be to remove the thumb from the right nostril and breathe out through the right nostril after left nostril is closed by the ring and little finger.
7. The second and the final step involves breathing in through the right nostril with left nostril still closed by the index and little finger. This will be followed by exhalation through the left nostril after removing the index and little finger and closing of the right nostril by thumb.

The above cycle of alternate nostrils breathing is to be continued at least for nine rounds in a single sitting with long, deep, smooth and effortless breath without application of any forces (with eyes closed).

Purification of the ida and pingala nadis and creation of the condition of equalized and balanced flow of prana through them to open the sushumna nadi is not an easy task as it apparently appears to be. The achievement of the goal requires hard work, consistent and persistent efforts under the active guidance of a Guru or teacher of proven credential. In this context it is to be kept in mind that nadis once purified does not necessarily remain purified forever; it can adversely get affected through bad food habits, negative thinking and lack of practice of the specific breathing process/processes.

With purification of the nadis and activation of sushumna, certain external signs appear on the person concerned. They are:-

1. lightness of the body,
2. brilliancy in complexion,
3. increase of the gastric fire,

4. leanness of the body,
5. absence of restlessness in the mind – body complex etc.

53. KUNDALINI SHAKTI

Divine consciousness or chaitanya is the universal prana or the vital energy (refer sections 21, 22 and 23 of part two). It is an auto energizing source of multifarious energy which is responsible for the creation, sustenance, destruction and recreation of all animated as well as inanimated objects in this universe. With respect to the mankind, this divine consciousness is known as chetana. Chetana is the energy required for the functioning of the human being. Depending on the types of activities performed, chetana is divided into two groups – active chetana and non active chetana. Extensive studies have revealed that active chetana constitutes 70 % of the vital energy or prana shakti in the human body and rest 30 % vital energy known as nonactive chetana lie dormant as kundalini shakti also known as spiritual energy.

Active chetana: It is the vital energy supplied to the gross body, mind, intellect and subtle ego. It moves through subtle nadis and chakras.

The non active chetana: The non active part of the vital energy lies dormant as Kundalini shakti at the base chakra mooladhara. The non-active chetana or kundalini shakti is used primarily for spiritual growth. It is not used for, nor does it take part in, day-to-day bodily functioning.

Non active chetana or kundalini shakti is present in every human being in a static and dormant form. It lies latent in the form of a serpent coiled three and a half times with face downward in the mooladhara chakra at the base of the spine.

Kundalini awakening happens either through spiritual practices or through spiritual transfer of energy.

54. AWAKENING OF KUNDALINI SHAKTI

It has been mentioned earlier that the journey from the physical to the spiritual level requires tremendous amount of energy. Awakening of kundalini shakti generates and provides this energy to a person for his movement from the physical plane to spiritual consciousness. There are two broad approaches to Kundalini awakening - active and passive.

The active approach involves systematic application of specific asana, breathing practices and meditation (to bring the mind to a state of thoughtlessness) all under the guidance of a competent teacher. Specific breathing practices in identified postures generate heat internally that sparks the kundalini shakti to awaken. When the kundalini shakti awakens, it hisses like a serpent beaten with a stick and moves upwards through the sushumna. This shakti passes through all the chakras and eventually unites with the supreme shiva shakti at the crown of the head leading to a person's spiritual enlightenment.

The passive approach called *shaktipat* refers to the bestowal of spiritual energy on one person by another. Generally it is the Guru (a spiritually evolved person) who bestows blessings to his disciple through shaktipat. *Shaktipat* can be transmitted with a sacred word or *mantra*, or by a look; it can also be transferred through thought or touch to the ajna chakra of the recipient. It is considered as an act of grace from the Guru to a deserving disciple. This transfer of energy itself initiates the awakening of the Kundalini shakti.

55. SPIRITUAL JOURNEY

Spiritual journey embraces carrying out specific breathing practices in identified postures associated with chanting of Guru mantras which help in the –

1. purification of the subtle nadis,
2. activation of the subtle chakras,

3. activation of the subtle sushumna,
4. awakening of the sleeping kundalini shakti,
5. rising of kundalini power through the chakras to meet with the supreme shiva shakti at the shahasrara.

With hard work and persistent effort, people in general can perceive and feel the above first three stages. To perceive and feel the fourth and achieve the fifth stage, resorting only to specific asana and breathing techniques is not enough; a person must also direct his whole life towards everything good. He has to cultivate a sattvik mind free from hatred, greed, anger, envy, jealousy, passion and dependency and live in love, harmony and understanding with the environment. It is only when the specific breathing practices in identified postures, chanting of mantras and the positive way of life (as mentioned above) merge with each other; a person makes progress in his journey towards spiritual consciousness.

To make a journey in the spiritual path, it is to be kept in mind that before the kundalini shakti is awakened, it must have its energy flow passageway and distributing centres in functioning orders. This necessitates that the sushumna and the chakras are awakened before the awakening of kundalini shakti. Between sushumna and the chakras, the chakras need to be awakened first so that the flow of sushumna once opened does not get interrupted. Flow of energy through sushumna gets arrested whenever it encounters a blocked chakra. The chakras therefore have to be awakened in the following sequence in order to ensure smooth ascent of the kundalini shakti (when awakened).

i. Mooladhara chakra.
ii. Swadhisthana chakra.
iii. Manipura chakra.
iv. Anahata chakra.
v. Vishudhi chakra
vi. Ajna chakra.

Once the above are ensured, awakened kundalini energy does not face any blockage in its journey upwards towards the shahasra chakra to get united with the shiva shakti . When this happens, a person is said to have attained spiritual consciousness.

The above however does not happen easily. It can take even several life times for a person to fully achieve spiritual consciousness. Even after awakening, the energy of kundalini may rise only up to manipura chakra and drop down to mooladhara chakra. It needs to be raised again and again through continuous efforts.

56. CONCLUSION

With the awareness and understanding of the breathing phenomenon, the activities involved in the act of breathing, different types of breathing practices, linkage between breath and emotion, a person understands that breathing can consciously and voluntarily be influenced to form a bridge between the conscious and unconscious areas of the mind- body complex. The mind and the body after all are not separate entities. The gross form of the mind is the body and the subtle form of the body is the mind. Once the above is realized, it helps a person to adapt appropriate breathing practices under different circumstances and situations to bring about overall improvements in the quality of his life.

With air, 'prana', the vital energy is also drawn into the body. Prana is more subtle than air or oxygen and is an auto energizing multifarious source of energy. It is through breathing that prana in the form of vayus gets distributed to different organs of the body, through subtle nadis and chakras. When the flows of the prana vayus are uninterrupted, a person enjoys healthy life. When the flow of prana through the nadis is interrupted or blocked for any reason, it results in pain associated with accumulation of toxin in the identified region of the body. These interruptions/blockages can be taken care of through specific breathing practices. Once the blockages are removed, smooth flow of prana is restored again with associated relief of pain and removal of toxins from the related areas of the physical system. Continuous practice of such breathing techniques clear all the blockages in the passageways of the prana vayus and purify them. Purification of the nadis is a pre-requisite for spiritual journey to commence. When the flow of prana through ida and pingala nadis are purified and become equal and balanced, sushumna nadi opens up signaling the commencement of spiritual journey. When the kundalini shakti is awakened through specific breathing practices, it's energy moves up the sushumna towards the shahasrara chakra for eventual achievement of divine consciousness.

Review of part one, part two and part three reveal that appropriate breathing practices have the power to

1. relieve all 'congestions' in the mind and body complex through improved blood circulation,
2. increase oxygen supply to brain and other parts of the body and ease the strain on the heart by increasing supply of oxygen to the heart,
3. enhance the detoxifying process,
4. decrease stress on organs of elimination and help the body to naturally cleanse and tonify,
5. increase vital energy and distribute it to various organs in different parts of the body,
6. lessen the stress responses by regulating the nervous system.
7. calm the mind from the clutch of the emotional state of disturbance/agitation/worry/anxiousness/fearfulness etc.
8. improve power of mental concentration and observation,
9. reverse the effects of stress related self-defeating habits,
10. strengthen coping skill,
11. produce relaxation and sense of inner self and inner power and enable a person to think and act courageously under pressure,
12. deepen meditation and spiritual connection,
13. increase awareness and managing capacity to balance subtle

energy systems affecting the physical, emotional, mental and spiritual bodies,

14. aid a person in spiritual journey for achieving divine consciousness.

Section 57, 58, 59 and 60 explain some of the terminologies which have been referred in different parts of the book.

57. FIVE BASIC ELEMENTS OF NATURE

It has been mentioned in section 53 of part three that divine consciousness or chaitanya, the universal prana is an auto energizing source of multifarious energy which is responsible for the creation, sustenance, destruction and recreation of all animated as well as inanimated objects in this universe. The animated and inanimated objects in this universe are all made up of the combination with the five elements of nature i.e. ether, water, fire, air and earth in varying degrees. Since these five elements originate from the subtle and all pervasive universal consciousness (divine power), traditionally they are worshipped as the embodiments of divinity. They are adored as the Goddess earth, various Goddesses representing rivers (water), the God of fire, the God of wind (air), and the God of ether (space).

Ether is the most subtle of the five elements and has its origin from 'divine consciousnesses'. It is less subtle than 'divine consciousnesses' or 'spirit'. Air has its origin from ether and is less subtle and pervasive than ether. Fire originates from air and is denser than air. Water has its origin from fire and is denser than fire. Earth has its origin from water and is the densest of the five elements. The density of the five elements increases from ether to air, to fire, to water, to earth.

The subtle energy which creates the 'objective elements' is called tanmatra. There are five tanmatras – shabda, sparsha, rupa, rasa and gandha. It is through the tanmatras that a person perceives the specific senses. Each element is related primarily to one tanmatra but can also contain a part of others as well. Ether comes out of tanmatra shabda (sound), air out of tanmatras shabda and sparsha (sound and touch), fire out of tanmatras shabda, sparsha, rupa (sound, touch, sight),water out of tanmatras shabda, sparsha, rupa and rasa (sound, touch, sight and taste) and earth out of the tanmatras shabda, sparsha, rupa, rasaand gandha (sound, touch,sight, taste and odour).

Each of the elements symbolically represent qualities and characteristics of matters as mentioned below:-

1. Earth does not necessarily mean soil only. Shape, form and stability represent the nature of earth. Anything and everything in nature that is heavy/solid /stable represents earth. It also represents highly restricted mobility. Element earth is also known as prithvi.
2. Water does not exclusively mean water only. Water represents anything and everything that is moist/cool/sticky and is able to act as both solvent and lubricant. It has the capacity to flow and move. Element water is also known as jal or apa.
3. Fire represents transformational energy which converts matter from one phase to another. Oxidation, chemical reaction and all forms of energy exchanges are represented by fire. It has the capacity to rise as well as spread in all directions. The element fire is also known as agni.
4. Air is representative of movement, fluidity and formlessness. It represents matter in gaseous form which is mobile, dynamic and subtle. It is lighter than fire and wafts about everywhere and is more pervasive than fire. The element air is also known as vayu or pavan.
5. Ether or space represents the nature of 'void'. It is lighter than air and is most unrestrained in its capacity to pervade. It represents the emptiness in which all other elements exist. It exists everywhere because sound energy pervades the entire creation. It is said that ether is the empty vastness of cosmos itself. Sound is the unique quality of space (ether). This element is also known as aakash.

Based on an individual characteristic, each of these elements have certain relationship with each other. As for example,

1. water and fire are repulsive to each other. They cannot coexist as they try to destroy each other. They have to be kept separated,
2. earth and water support and nurture each other. They can coexist,
3. water and air, fire and earth etc. are friendly and co operative towards each other, but given the first opportunity they separate out.

Laws of the nature are formed based on the relationship of these elements with respect to each other. Imbalance of these elements in nature leads to natural disaster.

The relevant representative nature and characteristics of the elements present in human body are mentioned below.

1. Earth: Bones, nails, muscles, tendon and ligaments are all earth like as are the walls of blood cells and body covering skin. Imbalance (less/excess) in the earth element leads to weakness, obesity, cholesterol, debility, low immunity, weight loss/weight gain, bones/muscular diseases etc.
2. Water: It occupies major volume in the form of different fluids like blood (carrier of oxygen), saliva, urine, semen, blood, sweat etc. It is the mover of nutrients and eliminator off waste products in human body. Imbalance in water element (less/excess) leads to cold, sinusitis, asthma, swellings, blood thinning or blood clotting, problem of urination, diseases of reproductive organs.
3. Fire represents hunger, thirst, sleep, etc. and is involved in oxidation, chemical reactions, metabolism and conversion of food to energy. Imbalance (less/excess) in fire element leads to skin diseases, increased coldness or heat in body, loss of vital energy, loss of appetite, indigestion, diabetes, and mental disorders.

4. Air: Represents running, walking, secretion of glands, contraction and expansion. It basically represents matter in gaseous form which is mobile, dynamic and subtle and exists without any form. It is also known as the element of movement and represents matter flowing freely and filling all empty spaces throughout the human body. All movements of the body and within the body, voluntary as well as involuntary, are effected by air element. It participates in all the biological functions and breathing phenomenon. It is also responsible for human thoughts, emotions, movement of electrical impulses along sensory nerves etc. Imbalance (less/excess) in air element leads to nervous disorders, blood pressure problems, lung disorders, physical pains, deformities, depression etc.
5. Some of the characteriscs of ether are love or attachment, jealousy or malice, shyness, fear, and passionate bonding. Cavities in nose, mouth, blood and lymph vessels, openings, pores in the intestinal tract and so forth which represent space (ether). It is the medium through which sound is transmitted, be it man made or otherwise. Imbalance (less/ excess) in space (ether) element leads to thyroid disorders, throat problems, speech disorders, epilepsy, madness, foolishness, ear diseases, etc.

Any disturbance in the balance of the five elements in the body causes manifestation of physical disorder. The five elements are associated with five human sensations, gnyanendriyas and karmendriyas.

58. THE FIVE HUMAN SENSATIONS

The five human sensations referred above are hearing, tasting, smelling, seeing and touching. They are the faculties which enable the mankind to perceive and experience anything and everything happening in this world.

Hearing: It is the sense through which a person distinguishes sound. The organ through which it functions is ear. Ear operates broadly through outer ear and inner ear. The outer ear consisting of cartilage and skin is visible from outside. It functions as a receptor and sends vibration to the inner ear via a tympanic membrane. The spiral shaped tubular inner ear converts the vibrations into sound and passes the message to the brain. The brain uses the sounds from both the ears and determines the distance and direction of sounds. Hearing enables a person to communicate his thoughts, intensions and desires to others.

Seeing: It is the sense which enables a person to distinguish objects in terms of beauty, size, shape, dimension etc. It functions through the eyes and enables a person to see objects and also to perceive passion and affection of others towards him. A person' eyes are on continuous work all the time till he goes to sleep. Eyes function like cameras – they take images of everything within the sight and immediately pass signals to the brain. The brain in turn instantly figures out what had been looked at.

Touching: It is the sense which enables a person to feel objects by the use of hands, feet and skin. It is the sense through which a person can feel the difference between soft and hard, smooth and rough, hot and cold and so forth. The sense of touch is spread throughout the entire body through nerves. Nerve endings (the part of the nerve that has the sensory receptors) on receipt of sensations relays the message to the brain for its immediate response. Finger tips have the maximum concentration of nerve endings.

Smelling: It is the sense which helps a person to identify objects through odours. Nose is the organ through which a person smells. Fumes of substances are the smell inputs. Inside the nose, there are mucous membranes which have smell receptors connected to a special nerve called olfactory nerve. On receipt of the fume molecules, the smell receptors react and send messages to the brain for its instant response. Different types of sensations identified by the sense of smelling are camphor, musk, flower, mint, ether, acrid, or putrid. Smelling also complements a person's ability to taste.

Tasting: It is the sense which helps a person to identify different tastes of substances. Taste buds are the receptors of taste sensation. They are the tiny sensory organs which appear mostly on the tongue, the roof of the mouth and in the back of the throat. In general taste buds:-

1. close to the tip of the tongue are sensitive to 'sweet taste',
2. in the back of the tongue are sensitive to 'bitter taste',
3. on the top of the tongue are sensitive to 'salty taste',
4. on the side of the tongue are sensitive to 'sour taste'.

The tongue also detects a sensation called umami from the taste receptors which are sensitive to amino acids. At the base of each taste bud there is a nerve that sends the sensations to the brain. Individual numbers of these taste buds vary from person to person. A person often comes across a terminology called mouth feel. Mouth feel is sensed by free nerve endings all over the inside of mouth and tongue. It focuses primarily on viscosity, temperature, burning, prickle, touch, pain etc. It is worthwhile to mention here that taste and flavor are distinctly different. While taste is a sense perceived by specialized receptor cells, flavor is a fusion of multiple senses. To perceive flavor, the brain interprets not only taste stimuli but also smell, tactile and thermal sensations.

Eyes, ears, nose, tongue and fingers are the sensing organs through which one sees, hears, smells, tastes, and feel touches respectively. Senses and sensing organs have separate identities. While the organs are physically existent, the senses are perceived. Perception can be explained as a human trait that enables a person to become aware of something through his organs of senses.

It is observed that when sleeping, a person cannot see anything (even if he sleeps with his eyes open), he cannot hear anything; in fact, he does not experience any sensation in sleep even though all his sensing organs are in order. It is further observed that even during waking hours, when a person's specific attention is withdrawn, his corresponding sense stops functioning; for example, when he looks at something while deeply thinking and concentrating on some other thing, he fails to notice people passing in front of him. This leads to the perception that senses do not function automatically; they function through the corresponding organs only when the specific senses are connected to the mind. This explains why

1. in deep sleep a person does not experience seeing, hearing etc. In deep sleep the mind and the senses are not connected, as a result the senses within remains non functional,
2. a person fails to notice people passing before him when he concentrates deeply on some other thing. In such a case the person's specific sense of seeing remains non functional as his mind is not connected to the sense of seeing, it is connected to 'some other thing'.

It is the senses through which thoughts are produced. Thoughts are produced when external stimuli (information from outside also called thought impulse) enter the mind through the organs of senses.

59. GNYANENDIYA/KARMENDRIYA

The sensations of hearing, feeling (feel of touch), seeing, tasting and smelling are perceived through the organs - ears, skin, eyes, tongue and nose respectively. These five organs through which one perceives the senses are called the organs of senses or gnyanendriyas. The word gnyanendriyas is derived from the combination of two sanskrit words gnyana (meaning knowledge or awareness of senses) and indriyas (meaning organs). The five gnyanendriyas are ears, skin, eyes, tongue and nose.

The organs through which the senses act upon and what they perceive are called organs of action or simply karmendriyas. The word karmendriya is derived from the combination of two kanskrit words karma (means work or action) and indriyas (means organs). The five karmendiyas vak (vocal cords/mouth), pani (hands), padam (feet), upastham (genitals) and payu (anus) act through speaking/eating, grasping/holding, walking/moving, procreating and eliminating respectively.

Each of the five elements is related to a karmendriya, a gnyanendriya, a tanmatra and a chakra as mentioned underneath.

Earth: Tanmatra related to earth is smell (odour or gandha). The gnanendriya is nose. Since it is through anus that the excretion of the waste matter back to the earth takes place, anus is considered to be the corresponding karmendriya. Mooladhara chakra connects to earth and gives stability to body and mind.

Water: is related to the perception of taste (rosa). Tanmatra related to water is taste. The corresponding gnynendriya is the tongue, but the karmendriya is the genitals. This is because the genitals are very closely linked to the tongue; without water neither genitals nor tongue can function properly. Swadhistana chakra is attuned with the water energy.

Fire: relates to vision because of its qualities of heat, light, and color. Related tanmatra is form (rupa) and gnyanendriya is eye. Fire's ability to give direction and impulse relates it to the feet (walking) as its karmendriya. Manipura chakra corresponds with the fire element.

Air: relates to the sense of touch. The related tanmatra is touch (sparsha).The related gnyanendriya is skin and the karmendriya is hand (holding). It corresponds to anahata chakra.

Space: is sound transmitting medium. It is functionally related to the sense of hearing. The related tanmatra is sound (shabda). The experience of space as luminous emptiness is the basis of higher spiritual consciousness. The gnyanendriya is ear. Since sound is produced through the vocal chord and mouth, these organs are considered to be the karmendriyas. Vishuddha chakra is directly related to the space element.

60. SATTVIK MIND

In the unmanifested universe, energy has three qualities, known as gunas - sattva, raja and tama. They exist together in equilibrium. Once energy takes form, one of these three qualities predominates. But no matter which quality prevails, an element of each of the other two gunas will always be present in that 'form'. Gunas exist in all beings (including human beings) in various degrees of concentration and combinations. Depending upon their relative strengths and combinations, they determine the nature of beings, its actions, behavior, attitude and its attachment to the objective world in which it lives.

Sattva guna is characterized by purity and knowledge. It is the most subtle or intangible of the three gunas and is nearest to divinity. Its predominance in a person is characterized by happiness, contentment, virtues like patience, perseverance, ability to forgive and be free from hatred, greed, anger, envy, jealousy, passion and dependency with spiritual yearning. With a sattvik mind a person lives in love, harmony and understanding with the environment. With prominence of sattva guna, a person lives and serves the society with no expectation of recognition or reward or any ulterior motive. Sattva guna dominated persons are known as sattavik.

Raja guna is characterized by action and passion. It plays significant role in activating the process of evolution based on the predominance of either of the balance two gunas. With prominence of raja guna, a person is more interested in personal gain and achievement. Raja guna dominated persons are known as rajasik

Tama guna is characterized by ignorance and inertia. Its predominance in a person is reflected by laziness, greed, attachment to worldly matters etc. With prominence of tama guna, to get moving ahead in life, a person has no hesitation to step on to other's toes or even harm the society. Tama Guna dominated persons are known as tamasik.

Prominence of the Gunas reflect on how people react to situations, make decisions, make choices and live their life. Hierarchically, tama is considered the lowest guna and sattva the highest guna. All material phenomena can be analysed in terms of the gunas. It is perceived that a person

1. influenced mainly by satta guna will be elevated to the heavenly planets at death,
2. influenced largely by Raja Guna will stay in human society,
3. infected with Tama Guna will enter into the lower species.

Only pure souls, transcending even Sattva guna, attain liberation and escape the entanglement of matter.

Review of the author's another book 'POWER OF THOUGHTS'

Harnessing Positivity

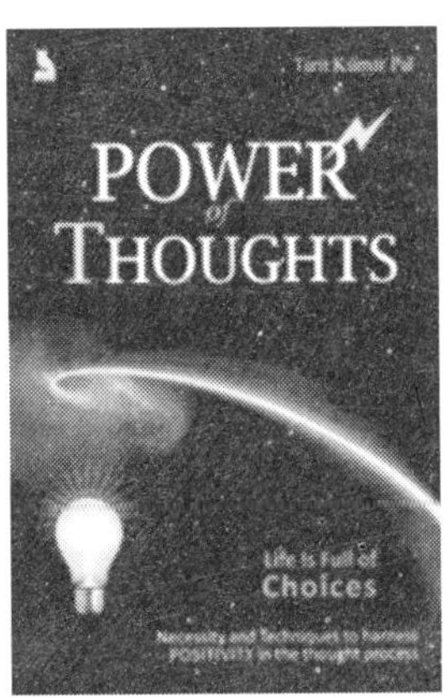

Tarit Kumar Pal
Pustak mahal
Page 168, INR 195

Power of Thoughts is an experiential guide written by Tarit Kumar Pal, a freelance consultant and a retired executive director from SAIL. Covering topics like decision-making, goal-setting, attitudinal conditioning and so on, it explores the many concerns people face in the course of their work life. It stresses upon the significance of thought energy, through the use of a number of practical techniques to manifest a life full of confidence and positivity. 'Life is full of choices', the tagline, forms the undercurrent of this first-person account by Pal.

His experiences of meeting positive and inspirational people, his articulation of his own beliefs, and the perseverance that helped him tide over the failures are interestingly conveyed.

Pal kindles the imagination by using a string of anecdotes to prove his points. His simple style and lack of pretension endear him to the readers. However, written essentially for corporate audience, there are many technical terms that might baffle a reader. Fortunately, a technical glossary has been provided at the end of the book. All in all, Power of Thoughts is a decent enough addition to the self-help basket of **Pustak Mahal.**

— **Life Positive**
(June 2014 Issue)

Comments on the book 'Power of Thoughts' by some of the readers

1. Heartiest congratulation on writing such an enlightening narrative.... I would ask my colleagues from Learning department to do a book reading session on your book with the associates.

   — C.P. Gurnani, CEO Mahindra Satyam and Managing Director Tech Mahindra.

2. The book is a very interesting read. Topics are covered in excellent order and many anecdotal examples are from real life Indian situations making it easier to relate to. We all have some knowledge on the topics taken up; the book converts this knowledge into understanding well.

   — Sanjiv Agarwal, Managing Director, MJR Steels, Kolkata.

3. I just completed reading your wonderful book. It is simply superb................ I feel it must be read and reread and should be suggested to friends to procure and read.

   — Gopikanta Ghosh. Author and former Joint Chief Executive Officer, Khadi and Village industries Commission, Mumbai.

4. "Many deviate from their path for lack of determination under pressure of unfavorable circumstances. Author has given many examples and also from his long executive career stressed the importance and impact of positive thoughts in building up successful career. A must read for all youths to build up strong thought process. This book will also help young executives in their decision making."

   — Dr. S.K. Dutta Choudhury, Rtd. Director. West Bengal Health Services.

5. The book is so much simpler and generalized that it will have wide spectrum of customers. I am sure it will be super hit and one of the best selling books.

   — Prof. Dr. S.K. Patel, Deptt. of Mech. Engg. National Institute of Technology, Rourkela.

6. The book Power of thoughts is very impressive and the contents have been explained nicely in co-relation with the title. Mr. Pal has expressed his own experience brilliantly and successfully explained the application of positive

thoughts in order to achieve success and also dealt in details about how to overcome hurdles of negative thoughts. The book has been written so nicely that anybody can understand it and I believe, people from all professions will be benefited from this book.

— Dr. Surojit Sinha, Associate Professor,
Indian Association for the cultivation of science, Kolkata

7. POWER OF THOUGHTS written by Mr. Tarit Kumar Pal from the personal experience is a step by step guide to develop positive attitude.

— Rati Kanta Ghosh, Managing Director,
Effluent & Water Treatment Engineers (P) Ltd, Kolkata .

8. .... The book is excellent. Though I had gone through it once, I want to go through it again many times in order to understand the core. The book is not meant only for budding managers but also for people in all walks of life and all cross section of the society, even for homemakers.

— C. Tarafdar, Patna

9. I admire you for your thought process and sharing your experience. I have shared the book with our marketing team............

— Shukhendu Bikash Misra,
Founder and Managing Director, MinexIndia, Mumbai.

10. We had bought 40 copies of your book from Pustak Mahal and presented to all General Managers and ED's of DSP. I enjoyed reading your book and found it very compelling. We are planning to buy another 100 copies for giving to our Management Trainees.

— Mrs. Reeta Banerjee, G.M (HRD) DSP, Durgapur, SAIL.
(Durgapur Steel Plant bought 101 copies more subsequently).

11. The book has been distributed among Sr. Officials of NMDC i.e GM and above. Overall response has been good and few officials told that the book is worth reading and useful for managers................

— Srinivasa Rao. NMDC Limited, Hyderabad.

12. Power of thoughts is a matured offering .Managing Change is depicted in a lucid manner .The reader enjoys the thought processing and the way to garner hidden talent without fear of attempting any new venture .Epilogue presents the spectrum of technical terms in an unique manner. A must read for the young and old generation.

— Jayanta & Binita Bagchi, Asansol